ICD-10-CM Preview

Anita C. Hazelwood, MLS, RHIA, FAHIMA
Carol A. Venable, MPH, RHIA

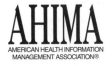

AHIMA
AMERICAN HEALTH INFORMATION
MANAGEMENT ASSOCIATION®

This book is based on ICD-9-CM as updated October 1, 2003, and the draft version of ICD-10-CM as posted on the National Center for Health Statistics Web site in June 2003.

ISBN 1-58426-120-X
AHIMA Product No. AC206003
Production No. IPC 2103-1500

Kathy Brouch, RHIA, CCS, Content Reviewer
Rita Scichilone, MHSA, RHIA, CCS, CCS-P, CHC, Content Reviewer
Marcia Loellbach, MS, Acquisitions Editor
Marcia Bottoms, Project Editor and Director of Publications

AHIMA strives to recognize the value of people from every racial and ethnic background as well as all genders, age groups, and sexual orientations by building its membership and leadership resources to reflect the rich diversity of the American population. AHIMA encourages the celebration and promotion of human diversity through education, mentoring, recognition, leadership, and other programs.

American Health Information Management Association
233 North Michigan Avenue, Suite 2150
Chicago, Illinois 60601-5800

http://www.ahima.org

Text Contents

About the Authors. iv
Foreword v
Preface ix
Introduction to ICD-10-CM 1
Chapter 1   Infectious and Parasitic Diseases. 27
Chapter 2   Neoplasms 35
Chapter 3   Diseases of the Blood and Blood-Forming Organs and
              Disorders of the Immune System. 41
Chapter 4   Endocrine, Nutritional, and Metabolic Diseases. 45
Chapter 5   Mental and Behavioral Disorders 51
Chapter 6   Diseases of the Nervous System 57
Chapter 7   Diseases of the Eye and Adnexa 63
Chapter 8   Diseases of the Ear and Mastoid Process. 67
Chapter 9   Diseases of the Circulatory System 71
Chapter 10   Diseases of the Respiratory System. 91
Chapter 11   Diseases of the Digestive System 97
Chapter 12   Diseases of the Skin and Subcutaneous Tissue. 103
Chapter 13   Diseases of the Musculoskeletal System and Connective Tissue 107
Chapter 14   Diseases of the Genitourinary System 115
Chapter 15   Conditions Related to Pregnancy and Childbirth 121
Chapter 16   Conditions Originating in the Perinatal Period 133
Chapter 17   Congenital Malformations, Deformations, and Chromosomal Abnormalities . 139
Chapter 18   Symptoms, Signs, and Abnormal Clinical and Laboratory Findings,
              Not Elsewhere Classified. 145
Chapter 19   Injury, Poisoning, and Other Consequences of External Causes. 151
Chapter 20   External Causes of Morbidity 161
Chapter 21   Factors Influencing Health Status and Contact with Health Services 169
Appendix   ICD-10-CM Coding Guidelines. 177
Index 251

CD-ROM Contents
ICD-10-CM Coding Guidelines
PowerPoint® Presentation
ICD-10-CM Fact Sheets

About the Authors

Carol A. Venable, MPH, RHIA, is a department head and professor at the University of Louisiana at Lafayette, and Anita C. Hazelwood, MLS, RHIA, FAHIMA, is an associate professor at the same university. They are the authors of *ICD-9-CM Diagnostic Coding and Reimbursement for Physician Services,* also published annually by the American Health Information Management Association.

Both authors have conducted numerous coding workshops at the local, state, and national levels. Moreover, they have published articles in the *Journal of AHIMA* and *Educational Perspectives in Health Information Management,* and they have served on the editorial review board of *Educational Perspectives in Health Information Management.* Active volunteers of AHIMA, Ms. Venable and Ms. Hazelwood are members of the Assembly on Education and the Coding Community of Practice. Both have served on the board of the Assembly on Education. Ms. Hazelwood also served on the board of the Society for Clinical Coding.

Foreword

The American Health Information Management Association (AHIMA) believes that adoption of the ICD-10-CM diagnostic classification system is imperative. Because ICD-9-CM is more than twenty years old, the system can no longer fulfill the need for accurate and complete healthcare data in the United States. In many areas, ICD-9-CM terminology and classifications are outdated and inconsistent with current medical practice. In addition, the system is rapidly running out of space and cannot accommodate the addition of new codes to address advances in medical knowledge or newly identified diseases. In some cases, proposals for new codes have not been implemented simply because there is insufficient space for a new code. ICD-9-CM codes also lack sufficient clinical detail to describe the severity or complexity of diagnoses, and the system does not provide sufficient codes for healthcare encounters for reasons other than treatment of disease or injury, such as preventive medicine.

The need for greater coding accuracy and specificity has increased considerably since the implementation of ICD-9-CM. The uses of coded data today go well beyond the purposes for which the ICD-9-CM coding system was designed in the 1970s. For example, coded data are now used for the following purposes:

- Measuring the quality, safety, and efficacy of healthcare services

- Making clinical decisions based on output from multiple systems

- Designing reimbursement systems and processing claims for payment

- Conducting research, epidemiological studies, and clinical trials

- Setting healthcare policy

- Designing healthcare delivery systems

- Monitoring resource utilization

- Improving clinical, financial, and administrative performance

- Identifying fraudulent and abusive practices

- Managing care and disease processes

- Tracking public health and health risks

- Providing information to consumers about the costs and outcomes of treatment options

Daily, healthcare entities (providers, payers, researchers, and other users) face problems that stem from the continued use of an obsolete classification system. For example:

- Providers are often required to submit additional documentation to support code assignments on reimbursement claims.

- The coding requirements of many payers conflict with official coding guidelines and with each other.

- Collecting complete and accurate data on medical conditions is difficult and time-consuming.

- Manual reviews of health records are sometimes required to meet the information needs of researchers and to fulfill other data mining functions.

- The lack of specificity in codes often leads to inconsistent code assignment.

- The potential for fraud and abuse is heightened because a variety of symptoms and medical conditions can be assigned to the same nonspecific code, which may or may not support medical necessity.

- Monitoring service and resource utilization, measuring performance, and analyzing healthcare costs and outcomes have become increasingly difficult with the ICD-9-CM system.

ICD-10-CM represents a significant improvement over ICD-9-CM. It incorporates much greater specificity and clinical detail, which would result in major improvements in the quality and usefulness of coded data. Most of the existing problems with ICD-9-CM would be addressed by the implementation of ICD-10-CM. ICD-10-CM provides much better information for nonacute care encounters, clinical decision making, and outcomes research. Medical advances that occurred since the implementation of ICD-9-CM have been incorporated into ICD-10-CM, as have the ICD-9-CM Coordination and Maintenance Committee's recommendations for new codes that could not be added to ICD-9-CM owing to space constraints.

Overall, the increased specificity in ICD-10-CM would result in the availability of better information, which, in turn, would:

- Improve the ability of providers, payers, government agencies, and others to measure the quality, safety, and efficacy of healthcare services

- Support providers' and payers' performance improvement activities

- Improve public health surveillance

- Enhance health policy decision making

- Improve the ability of payers to forecast the healthcare needs of their beneficiaries and to trend and analyze healthcare costs

- Reduce payers' and providers' costs due to the ability to effectively monitor service and resource utilization, analyze healthcare costs, monitor outcomes, measure performance, and detect fraud and abuse

- Allow appropriate refinements of reimbursement systems to better reflect the actual cost of patient care

- Improve the ability of providers and payers to negotiate reimbursement rates

- Reduce the need for manual review of health records to support reimbursement claims and to perform research and data mining

The Health Insurance Portability and Accountability Act (HIPAA) of 1996 mandated federal regulations on electronic healthcare transactions and code sets. Under HIPAA, the adoption of any new coding system, including ICD-10-CM, as a national standard must incorporate the following features:

- Public hearings with testimony from various stakeholders and solicitation of public comments

- Recommendation for adoption by the National Committee on Vital and Health Statistics (NCVHS) to the Secretary of Health and Human Services (HHS)

- Publication of a Notice of Proposed Rule-Making in the *Federal Register,* with opportunity for public submission of comments

- Publication of a final rule with implementation date in the *Federal Register*

Although the continued use of ICD-9-CM as the standard diagnostic code set threatens to limit the U.S. healthcare industry's ability to collect and use healthcare data effectively, the implementation date for ICD-10-CM has not yet been determined. At the time this publication went to press, the NCVHS was scheduled to hold a meeting on September 23 and 24, 2003, to discuss a report prepared by the Rand Corporation on the costs and benefits of adopting and implementing ICD-10-CM as a replacement for ICD-9-CM. The report also considers the costs and benefits of implementing the *International Classification of Diseases, Tenth Revision, Procedure Coding System* (ICD-10-PCS). The results of the meeting will be published in the *Federal Register,* at http://www.access.gpo.gov//su_docs/fedreg/a03079c.html and at http://www.ncvhs.hhs.gov.

The AHIMA and other healthcare associations including the American Hospital Association and the American Medical Association hope that the NCVHS will decide to recommend adoption of ICD-10-CM and ICD-10-PCS to the Secretary of Health and Human Services during the fall of 2003.

Sue Prophet-Bowman, RHIA, CCS
Director of Coding Policy and Compliance
American Health Information Management Association

September 2003

Preface

This *ICD-10-CM Preview* is based on the revised draft of ICD-10-CM as published by the National Center for Health Statistics (NCHS) in June 2003 and on ICD-9-CM as updated for October 1, 2003. The June 2003 draft of ICD-10-CM is available on the Centers for Disease Control Web site. Because the system is in the public domain, the complete draft can be downloaded electronically, printed, reproduced, or viewed from the Web site at www.cdc.gov/nchs/about/otheract/icd9/icd10.htm. The June 2003 draft includes revisions in the May 2002 draft suggested by the public. Two items that were not previously published—the ICD-10-CM official coding guidelines and the Table of Drugs and Chemicals—also became available on the Web site in June 2003. The Web site is the best source for the most current version of the codes in the revised classification system.

The American Health Information Management Association (AHIMA) used the June 2003 draft in its ICD-10-CM testing project, which was conducted during the summer of 2003. Results from the testing will be submitted to the NCHS for use in assessing the utility and functionality of ICD-10-CM and its related rules and guidelines. A cost–benefit analysis of implementing ICD-10-CM and ICD-10-PCS (the new procedural coding system) in the United States was also conducted during the summer of 2003. A final decision on the adoption of ICD-10-CM and the timing of implementation will probably be made by the end of 2003.

The *ICD-10-CM Preview* is a perfect introduction to the revised classification system for clinical coding professionals, health information managers, clinicians, information systems professionals, administrators, consultants, software vendors, and third-party payers. This practical overview provides enough information to address most potential issues during the planning stage and thus make ICD-10-CM implementation a manageable process.

The *ICD-10-CM Preview* includes information that is presented in three different formats. The printed portion of the book can be used by individuals who are interested in learning about ICD-10-CM diagnostic coding or are charged with planning for ICD-10-CM implementation. The text includes an index and an appendix that reproduces the NCHS's official coding guidelines for ICD-10-CM. The CD-ROM included at the back of the book offers similar information in two additional formats: PowerPoint® slides and Word®-based fact sheets, all of which may be customized for specific audiences or organizations. For example, the slide presentation could be used as the basis for in-service education of clinicians, and the fact sheets could be distributed to attendees as handouts that attendees could refer to after the in-service session is over. A PDF version of the official coding guidelines is also included on the CD-ROM at the back of the book.

The *ICD-10-CM Preview* is made up of two parts. The introduction covers the historical background of the classification system, the differences between ICD-9-CM and ICD-10-CM, the structure and characteristics of ICD-10-CM, and the implementation of ICD-10-CM. The second part provides a chapter-by-chapter analysis of the changes made in the ICD-9-CM system to create the ICD-10-CM system. Readers should note that the codes provided as examples may not be complete and that the Web version of ICD-10-CM is the most current and up-to-date resource for actual codes.

Introduction to ICD-10-CM

The clinical modification of the *International Classification of Diseases, Ninth Revision* (ICD-9-CM), has been used in the United States for morbidity and mortality reporting and indexing since 1979. However, the system has become increasingly out-of-date since the implementation of the Health Insurance Portability and Accountability Act (HIPAA) in 2003. ICD-9-CM cannot meet all the requirements of the HIPAA standards, especially in the areas of electronic transactions and code sets.

Initially, ICD-9-CM codes were designed for the purpose of disease indexing in the hospital inpatient setting. They were not intended to be used in reimbursement systems and were not used for this purpose until the implementation of the Medicare prospective payment system in 1983.

Today, the various prospective payment systems being used for healthcare reimbursement require meticulous health record documentation, advanced coding skills, and high levels of data quality. To meet these requirements, transitioning to the use of the tenth revision of *International Classification of Diseases and Related Health Problems* (ICD-10) is currently being proposed. A clinical modification of ICD-10 has been designed as a replacement classification system for ICD-9-CM to be used in the United States. The clinical modification of ICD-10 was created specifically to address the deficiencies in ICD-9-CM and to enhance the quality of administrative data available in the United States.

Coded data are used in a number of ways, namely:

- For designing claims-processing systems specifically for reimbursement purposes

- For measuring the safety, quality, and efficacy of medical care

- For designing healthcare delivery systems and setting healthcare policy

- For monitoring the utilization of resources and improving the financial, clinical, and administrative performance of healthcare organizations

- For providing healthcare consumers with data on the cost and outcomes of various treatment options

- For identifying, tracking, and managing public health risks and disease processes

- For recognizing and identifying abusive or fraudulent reimbursement practices and trends

- For conducting healthcare research and clinical trials and participating in epidemiological studies

It has become obvious that to fulfill all these requirements, a classification system that provides greater coding accuracy and specificity is greatly needed.

History of Classification Systems

From a foundation based on the work of the physician Hippocrates, the early Greeks made the first attempts to group health-related data on the basis of disease processes. But it was not until the seventeenth century that Captain John Graunt, a London physician, directed the world's attention to the various causes of mortality (death) and morbidity (illness). Graunt's publication, *The London Bills of Mortality,* marked the first real attempt to study disease processes from a statistical point of view.

The history of statistical healthcare classification systems dates back to as early as the eighteenth century, when in 1837 William Farr worked to develop a better system for disease classification and international uniformity in the use of health-related statistics. Farr's classification of diseases by anatomical site served as the basis for the *International List of Causes of Death,* which ultimately served as the foundation for the current international system of collecting vital statistics.

In 1893, Dr. Jacques Bertillon developed the *Bertillon Classification of Causes of Death.* Five years later, in 1898, the American Public Health Association (APHA) recommended that Bertillon's classification system be adopted for use in Canada, Mexico, and the United States. The APHA also recommended that the classification system be revised every ten years. Subsequent revisions, entitled the *International Classification of Causes of Death,* were completed in 1900, 1910, 1920, 1929, and 1938. During this period of time, the classification was used only to classify causes of mortality.

That changed, however, in 1948, when the World Health Organization (WHO) published the sixth revision of the classification. For the first time, the revision also included lists for the tabulation of information on morbidity. Along with this sixth revision, a recommendation was made that governments establish national committees on health and vital statistics to coordinate all statistical activities in their respective countries and at the same time to serve as a link to the WHO.

Modern Classification Systems

In the late 1950s, the U.S. Public Health Service published a modification of the seventh revision of ICD as the *International Classification of Diseases, Adapted for Indexing Hospital Records by Diseases and Operations* (ICDA). ICDA was used as a tool for the indexing of diseases treated in hospitals. Modifications to the ICDA were made in 1962 to provide greater detail and to introduce a classification of surgical operations.

Because even greater detail and specificity were needed in the United States, the eighth revision of the classification, the *International Classification of Diseases, Adapted for Use in the United States,* was published in 1968. This publication served as the basis for coding morbidity and mortality statistics in the United States and served as a method of indexing all diagnoses and operative procedures in hospital records until 1979.

The ninth revision of the *International Classification of Diseases* was published in 1977 as the *International Classification of Diseases, Ninth Revision* (ICD-9). Two years later, in 1979, the WHO adopted ICD-9 as its system for statistical classification. ICD-9 became a universal system for the grouping of illnesses and was used secondarily as the foundation of hospital disease indexing.

In 1977, the National Center for Health Statistics, a division of the U.S. Centers for Disease Control, began to develop a modification of ICD-9 to be used primarily in the United States. This system is known as the *International Classification of Diseases, Ninth Revision, Clinical Modification* (ICD-9-CM). Since 1979 there have been numerous changes and revisions to the ICD-9-CM system, and ICD-9-CM is still being in the United States used today.

Guidelines for ICD-9-CM coding are developed by four organizations, collectively called the Cooperating Parties. These organizations are the American Hospital Association (AHA), the American Health Information Management Association (AHIMA), the Centers for Medicare and Medicaid Services (CMS), and the National Center for Health Statistics (NCHS). The Cooperating Parties began their relationship in the 1980s. Together they are responsible for developing official coding guidelines as well as for ensuring the proper application of the ICD-9-CM system.

Each of the four organizations has specific responsibilities in maintaining and updating ICD-9-CM. The NCHS maintains the disease classification, and the CMS maintains the procedure classification. To help in the process of maintenance, the ICD-9-CM Coordination and Maintenance Committee reviews all official updates to the coding system. The meetings of the Coordination and Maintenance Committee are open for input from interested parties. The AHA sponsors the Central Office on ICD-9-CM and publishes *Coding Clinic,* the source of the official coding guidelines for ICD-9-CM. The AHIMA provides coding education and certifies professional coders. All four Cooperating Parties must approve any new or revised coding guidelines.

The WHO owns and publishes the international version of the ICD classification system. In 1992, the WHO published the tenth revision of the ICD system, which is now being used by many countries. The goal of the tenth revision was to expand the content, purpose, and scope of the system. It was designed to include ambulatory care services, increase clinical detail, capture risk factors in primary care, identify emergent diseases, and develop group diagnoses for epidemiological purposes.

Subsequently, the United States developed, but has not yet implemented, a clinical modification of the tenth revision of the ICD system. The NCHS began the first round of testing for the system in 1997. The AHIMA has tested the June 2003 version of ICD-10-CM, and the CMS has conducted a cost–benefit study to quantify the value of implementing the new system in the United States. The final version of ICD-10-CM will not be released until all adjustments have been made and the coding guidelines have been finalized. Although the United States began using ICD-10 in 1999 to classify mortality statistics, ICD-10-CM probably will not be implemented until October 2005 at the earliest.

Comparison of ICD-10-CM with ICD-9-CM

The purpose of the *International Classification of Diseases* classification system is to promote international agreement on the collection, classification, processing, and presentation of health data, including both mortality and morbidity data, so that health data from around the world can be meaningfully compared. In everyday practice, ICD has become an international diagnostic classification system used for all general epidemiological and healthcare purposes. Because the United States is required to report mortality and morbidity data to the WHO under an agreement that is similar to an international treaty, any revisions made to the tenth revision of the system must conform to ICD-10 conventions. As owner and publisher of ICD-10, the WHO promotes the development of any adaptations that will expand the usefulness and comparability of health statistics. Therefore, the WHO has authorized an adaptation of ICD-10 (ICD-10-CM) for use in the United States.

Benefits of ICD-10-CM

Compared to ICD-9-CM, ICD-10-CM codes generally provide greater specificity and more clinical information as well as additional information relevant to ambulatory and managed care encounters. In addition, the structure of ICD-10-CM allows for the possibility of greater expansion in the code system. ICD-10-CM also extends beyond the simple classification of diseases and injuries to include health-related risk factors that are frequently encountered in the primary care setting. The new system also includes diseases identified since the most recent revision of ICD-9-CM.

General terminology, as well as the disease classification itself, has been updated to be consistent with accepted and current clinical practice. The expanded degree of specificity should provide more detailed information to assist providers, payers, and policy makers in establishing appropriate reimbursement rates, improving the delivery of healthcare, improving and evaluating the overall quality of patient care, and effectively monitoring both service and resource utilization.

Brief Comparison of ICD-10-CM with ICD-9-CM

ICD-10-CM was designed to offer significant advantages over ICD-9-CM. The changes should result in significant improvements in both the quality and the usefulness of data for various healthcare settings.

General changes in the content and the format of ICD-10-CM include the following:

- The hierarchical structure is the same for both classification systems, but ICD-10-CM codes are alphanumeric and include all letters except U, which is reserved for new diseases of uncertain etiology.

- ICD-9-CM's V and E codes are incorporated into the main classification in ICD-10-CM.

- ICD-10-CM codes can be as long as seven characters; ICD-9-CM's longest codes include five characters.

- ICD-10-CM incorporates additional information related to ambulatory and managed care encounters.

- Conditions that were not uniquely identified in ICD-9-CM have been assigned code numbers in ICD-10-CM.

- In ICD-10-CM, as in ICD-9-CM, some three-character categories are left vacant to allow for code revisions and future additions.

- In contrast to ICD-9-CM, which classifies injuries by type (sprain, fracture, dislocation, and so on), ICD-10-CM groups injuries first by site (arm, leg, ankle, and so on) and then by type.

- Expanded *excludes* notes provide guidance on the hierarchy of the chapters and clarify priority of code assignment or "special group" chapters.

- Some conditions with new treatment protocols or recently discovered or new etiology are listed in more appropriate chapters.

In addition, ICD-10-CM offers several new or expanded features, including the following:

- Combination codes are used for both symptom and diagnosis and etiology and manifestations (for example, K50.013, Crohn's disease of small intestine with fistula).

- Many codes have been expanded, particularly in the neoplasm and injury chapters, to include laterality (for example, C56.0, Malignant neoplasm of right ovary).

- Classifications that indicate a patient's trimester are included in the obstetrics chapter (for example, O60.2, Preterm labor, second trimester).

- In the section on diabetes, codes are included for types that require insulin therapy and types that do not.

- Codes for postoperative complications have been expanded, and a distinction is made between intraoperative complications and postprocedural disorders (for example, K91, Intraoperative and postprocedural complications and disorders of digestive system, NEC).

Types of Code Changes

In general, most of the differences between ICD-10-CM and ICD-9-CM are of the following types:

- *Grouping of codes:* Conditions have been grouped in a more logical fashion than in ICD-9-CM. In many cases, this improvement was accomplished by moving conditions from one chapter to another or one section to another. Numerous codes have been added to, deleted from, combined, or moved in ICD-10-CM. ICD-10-CM includes four more chapters than ICD-9-CM, although the conditions classified to the additional chapters in ICD-10-CM are not necessarily new, and most were classified to other chapters in ICD-9-CM.

- *More complete descriptions:* In ICD-10-CM, the subcategory titles are usually complete so that the coding professional does not have to read previous codes to understand the meaning of the code.

- *Fifth and sixth characters:* Fifth and sixth characters are incorporated into the code listing rather than having common fifth characters listed at the beginning of a chapter, section, or category.

- *Laterality:* ICD-10-CM incorporates laterality of conditions or injuries at the fifth- or sixth-character level.

- *Increased specificity:* ICD-10-CM offers greatly expanded detail for the various conditions. Many categories that were limited to three or four digits in ICD-9-CM have fifth, sixth, and even seventh characters, or extensions, in ICD-10-CM. In some cases, single ICD-9-CM codes were split into several ICD-10-CM codes to provide greater specificity.

- *Use of extensions:* Extensions are used in ICD-10-CM to provide additional information. They are most often found in the injury codes but also are found in other chapters.

- *Combination codes:* Numerous codes in ICD-10-CM group etiology and manifestation. In ICD-9-CM, generally two codes are required to code etiology and manifestation.

- *Terminology used:* Many of the category code/subcategory code titles have been changed to reflect new technology and more recent medical terminology.

- *Postprocedural conditions:* Many more codes have been added to ICD-10-CM to describe postoperative or postprocedural conditions.

- *Trimester specificity:* ICD-10-CM codes in the pregnancy, delivery, and puerperium chapter include those designating the trimester in which the condition occurs.

- *New codes:* ICD-10-CM provides codes for many conditions that were not included in ICD-9-CM, most notably, codes for blood type and alcohol level.

The increased specificity of the ICD-10-CM codes will make complete and accurate documentation increasingly important after the new system is implemented. Health information managers and coding professionals will need to help radiologists, pathologists, and other physicians and clinicians become more aware of documentation requirements.

Health record forms and/or computer fields may need to be reviewed and revised to incorporate the data needed to assign codes or process coded data. This review of forms and/or computer fields should begin many months prior to ICD-10-CM implementation.

More information specific to each ICD-10-CM chapter is discussed later in this book. Obviously, however, every change could not be discussed in detail, and the information provided is based on the preliminary version of ICD-10-CM that was available when this book was written.

General Structure and Characteristics of ICD-10-CM

The tenth revision of the *International Statistical Classification of Diseases and Related Health Problems* is organized in three volumes. Volume 1 is a tabular list of the alphanumeric codes that represent diagnoses. Volume 2 explains the rules and guidelines for assigning ICD-10 codes, and Volume 3 is an index to the codes in the Tabular List. Currently, ICD-10-CM, the clinical modification of ICD-10 created for use in the United States, includes only in two volumes, the Tabular List and the Alphabetic Index. It has not yet been decided whether a modification of ICD-10 volume 2 will be included in the final version of ICD-10-CM.

Tabular List

Like the first volume of ICD-9-CM, the first part of ICD-10-CM is structured as a multichapter tabular list that follows specific conventions. The conventions pertain to the punctuation, abbreviations, and terminology used to guide users in the assignment of appropriate diagnostic codes from the classification.

Structure of the Tabular List

The ICD-10-CM Tabular List is divided into twenty-one chapters. Although anatomy is the primary axis of classification in most of the chapters, several chapters are arranged by etiology (neoplasms, for example) or other criteria (external causes, for example).

The chapters of the ICD-10-CM classification system include:

1. Certain infectious and parasitic diseases (A00–B99)

2. Neoplasms (C00–D48)

3. Diseases of the blood and blood-forming organs and certain disorders involving the immune mechanism (D50–D89)

4. Endocrine, nutritional and metabolic diseases (E00–E90)

5. Mental and behavioral disorders (F01–F99)

6. Diseases of the nervous system (G00–G99)

7. Diseases of the eye and adnexa (H00–H59)

8. Diseases of the ear and mastoid process (H60–H95)

9. Diseases of the circulatory system (I00–I99)

10. Diseases of the respiratory system (J00–J99)

11. Diseases of the digestive system (K00–K93)

12. Diseases of the skin and subcutaneous tissue (L00–L99)

13. Diseases of the musculoskeletal system and connective tissue (M00–M99)

14. Diseases of the genitourinary system (N00–N99)

15. Pregnancy, childbirth and the puerperium (O00–O99)

16. Certain conditions originating in the perinatal period (P00–P96)

17. Congenital malformations, deformations and chromosomal abnormalities (Q00–Q99)

18. Symptoms, signs and abnormal clinical and laboratory findings, not elsewhere classified (R00–R99)

19. Injury, poisoning and certain other consequences of external causes (S00–T98)

20. External causes of morbidity (V01–Y98)

21. Factors influencing health status and contact with health services (Z00–Z99)

The first character of the ICD-10-CM code is a capital letter, and each letter is associated with a particular chapter, except for the letters D and H. The letter D is used in both chapter 2, Neoplasms, and chapter 3, Diseases of the blood and blood-forming organs and certain disorders involving the immune mechanism. The letter H is used in both chapters 7, Diseases of the eye and adnexa, and 8, Diseases of the ear and mastoid process. Four chapters (1, 2, 9, and 10) include codes that begin with more than one letter in the first position. To allow for future revisions or expansions of the classification, every available code is not used.

Chapters are divided into blocks made up of three-character categories that cover similar or closely related conditions. Each chapter in the Tabular List of ICD-10-CM begins with a summary of the blocks to provide an overview of the codes in the chapter. For example:

Chapter 3

Diseases of the blood and blood-forming organs and certain disorders involving the immune mechanism (D50–D89)

This chapter contains the following blocks:

D50–D53   Nutritional anemias
D55–D59   Hemolytic anemias
D60–D64   Aplastic and other anemias
D65–D69   Coagulation defects, purpura and other hemorrhagic conditions
D70–D78   Other diseases of blood and blood-forming organs
D80–D89   Certain disorders involving the immune mechanism

The three-character categories (sometimes referred to as rubrics) are the backbone of the coding system. The disease classification system begins with category A00 and ends with category Z99, although not all letters of the alphabet or all the numbers possible in the classification have been used in the current version of the classification.

A three-character category may represent a single disease entity (generally based on frequency or severity) or a group of closely related conditions. For example:

D51   Vitamin B$_{12}$ deficiency anemia
D53   Other nutritional anemias

The classification usually provides codes for other and unspecified conditions. For example:

D89   Other disorders involving the immune mechanism, not elsewhere classified

K46   Unspecified abdominal hernia

Although most three-character categories are further divided into four-character subcategories, some three-character categories have not been subdivided because additional specificity is not needed. For example:

O76   Abnormality in fetal heart rate and rhythm complicating labor and delivery

P90   Convulsions of newborn

R64   Cachexia

Four- or five-character subcategories generally classify the disease by one of several axes such as etiology (for example, staphylococcal), anatomic site (for example, upper quadrant), or severity (for example, acute). In general, the next-to-the-last subdivision is identified by a fourth-character 8 placed after a decimal point (.8), which is used to indicate some "other" specified category when a condition does not warrant its own subdivision. The last four-character subcategory (fourth-character .9) is usually reserved for an unspecified condition, which means that not enough information is available to code to a more specific condition. Thus, the decimal digits 8 and 9 are generally reserved for other and unspecified subcategories. For example:

P51   Umbilical hemorrhage of newborn
    P51.0   Massive umbilical hemorrhage of newborn
    P51.8   Other umbilical hemorrhages of newborn
            Slipped umbilical ligature NOS
    P51.9   Umbilical hemorrhage of newborn, unspecified

O11   Pre-existing hypertensive disorder with superimposed proteinuria
      O11.1   Pre-existing hypertensive disorder with superimposed proteinuria, first trimester
      O11.2   Pre-existing hypertensive disorder with superimposed proteinuria, second trimester
      O11.3   Pre-existing hypertensive disorder with superimposed proteinuria, third trimester
      O11.9   Pre-existing hypertensive disorder with superimposed proteinuria, unspecified trimester

Subcategories may be further subdivided into five- and six-character codes to provide even greater specificity or additional information about the condition being coded. For example:

A39   Meningococcal infection
      A39.5   Meningococcal heart disease
            A39.50   Meningococcal carditis, unspecified
            A39.51   Meningococcal endocarditis
            A39.52   Meningococcal myocarditis
            A39.53   Meningococcal pericarditis

      O10.3   Pre-existing hypertensive heart and renal disease complicating pregnancy, childbirth and the puerperium
            O10.31   Pre-existing hypertensive heart and renal disease complicating pregnancy
                  O10.311   Pre-existing hypertensive heart and renal disease complicating pregnancy, first trimester
                  O10.312   Pre-existing hypertensive heart and renal disease complicating pregnancy, second trimester
                  O10.313   Pre-existing hypertensive heart and renal disease complicating pregnancy, third trimester
                  O10.319   Pre-existing hypertensive heart and renal disease complicating pregnancy, unspecified trimester
            O10.32   Pre-existing hypertensive heart and renal disease complicating childbirth

      P03.8   Newborn (suspected to be) affected by other specified complications of labor and delivery
            P03.81   Newborn (suspected to be) affected by abnormality in fetal (intrauterine) heart rate or rhythm
                Excludes 1:   neonatal cardiac dysrhythmia (P29.1)
                P03.810   Newborn (suspected to be) affected by abnormality in fetal (intrauterine) heart rate or rhythm before the onset of labor
                P03.811   Newborn (suspected to be) affected by abnormality in fetal (intrauterine) heart rate or rhythm during labor
                P03.819   Newborn (suspected to be) affected by abnormality in fetal (intrauterine) heart rate or rhythm, unspecified as to time of onset

When a category has been subdivided into four-, five-, or six-character codes, the code assigned must represent the highest level of specificity represented in the classification. This means that when a three-character category is not further subdivided, the category may be assigned as a code, but when a category is subdivided into subcategory codes, one of the subcategory codes must be assigned. For example, when a four-character subcategory has been subdivided, the four-character code cannot stand alone because it is considered an invalid code. Therefore, in the preceding examples, A39.5, O10.3, and P03.81 are considered invalid codes.

Five- and six-character codes are presented in their natural sequence under the appropriate four- or five-character codes. This format is different from the format in ICD-9-CM, where five-character codes could appear at the beginning of a chapter or subchapter.

ICD-10-CM sometimes uses dummy placeholders for future additions to the classification. The dummy is always a lowercase letter ex (*x*). The poisoning codes (T36–T50) and toxic effects codes (T51–T65) are the best examples of the use of dummy *x,* which occurs as the fifth character in six-character codes.

ICD-10-CM uses extensions in many categories to provide additional information. Extensions are always the seventh and final character in a code. When the code contains fewer than seven characters, dummy *x* placeholders are added to fill out the empty characters. Examples of categories and subcategories that require extensions include the following:

V45   Car occupant injured in collision with railway train or railway vehicle
The following 7th character extensions are to be added to each code from category V45:
    a   initial encounter
    d   subsequent encounter
    q   sequela
    V45.0   Car driver injured in collision with railway train or railway vehicle in nontraffic accident

R40.2   Coma
Coma NOS
Unconsciousness NOS
Code first any associated:
    coma in fracture of skull (S02.–)
    coma in intracranial injury (S06.–)
The following 7th character extensions are to be added to codes R40.21, R40.22, R40.23:
    1   in the field [EMT or ambulance]
    2   at arrival to emergency department
    3   at hospital admission
    4   24 hours after hospital admission
    9   unspecified time

S74   Injury of nerves at hip and thigh level
Code also any associated open wound (S71.–)
Excludes 2:   injury of nerves and ankle and foot level (S94.–)
                    injury of nerves at lower leg level (S84.–)
The following 7th character extensions are to be added to each code for category S74:
    a   initial encounter
    d   subsequent encounter
    q   sequela

S79   Other and unspecified injuries of hip and thigh
The following 7th character extensions are to be added to each code for subcategories S79.0 and S79.1:
A fracture not designated as open or closed should be coded to closed.

    a   initial encounter for fracture
    d   subsequent encounter for fracture with routine healing
    g   subsequent encounter for fracture with delayed healing
    j   subsequent encounter for fracture with nonunion
    m   subsequent encounter for fracture with malunion
    q   sequela

The appropriate selection of an extension depends directly on documentation provided by the patient's physician. Physicians should be advised to include the required documentation in patients' health records so that coding professionals have enough information to select the correct extensions.

Conventions Followed in the Tabular List

To correctly assign ICD-10-CM diagnoses, users must understand certain conventions used in the classification. Just as in ICD-9-CM, abbreviations, punctuation, symbols, and notes have special meanings that affect code assignment.

Punctuation

The different types of punctuation included in ICD-10-CM include square brackets, colons, parentheses, and the point dash.

Square brackets are used to enclose synonyms, alternative wordings, and explanatory phrases. For example:

B00   Herpesviral [herpes simplex] infections

F41.0   Panic disorder [episodic paroxysmal anxiety] without agoraphobia

The colon is used with **includes** or **excludes** statements in which the words that precede the statements are not considered complete terms and therefore must be modified by one of the words indented under the statement before the condition can be assigned to that code. For example:

D00   Carcinoma in situ of oral cavity, esophagus and stomach
    D00.0   Carcinoma in situ of lip, oral cavity and pharynx
        Excludes 1:   carcinoma in situ of aryepiglottic fold or interarytenoid fold,
            laryngeal aspect (D02.0)
            carcinoma in situ of epiglottis:
                NOS (D02.0)
                suprahyoid portion (D02.0)

Parentheses are used in the Tabular List in several important situations. First, they are used to enclose supplementary words that may be present or absent in the statement of diagnosis without affecting the code assignment. Terms in parentheses are considered nonessential modifiers. For example:

I10   Essential (primary) hypertension
    Includes: high blood pressure
              hypertension (arterial) (benign) (essential) (malignant) (primary) (systemic)

O35.6   Maternal care for (suspected) damage to fetus by radiation

In the first example, the terms in parentheses do not have to be present in the diagnostic statement in order to use code I10. Similarly, the code in the second example may be used whether damage is suspected or confirmed.

Parentheses also are used to enclose the code or codes to which an **excludes** term refers. For example:

A40   Streptococcal sepsis
    Excludes 1:   neonatal (P36.0–P36.1)
              puerperal sepsis (O85)
              sepsis due to Streptococcus, group D (A41.81)

Finally, parentheses are used at the beginning of a chapter to enclose the range of three-character codes included in that chapter. Similarly, parentheses are used at the block or subcategory level to indicate the codes included in that block. For example:

Chapter 1
Certain infectious and parasitic diseases (A00–B99)

The point dash is used primarily in **excludes** notes to remind the user that a fourth character exists and that the Tabular List should be referenced to find the appropriate character. For example:

J16 Pneumonia due to other infectious organisms, not elsewhere classified
Code first any associated lung abscess (J85.1)
Excludes 1: congenital pneumonia (P23.–)
ornithosis (A70)
pneumocystosis (B59)
pneumonia NOS (J18.9)

P59 Neonatal jaundice from other and unspecified causes
Excludes 1: jaundice due to inborn errors of metabolism (E70–E90)
kernicterus (P57.–)

Words and Phrases with Special Meanings

The word *and* always means *and/or* when used in narrative statements. When the words *with* and *without* represent the options for the final character in a set of codes, the option representing *without* should be assumed unless the documentation supports the assignment of a *with* code. In five-character codes, a zero used as the last character represent *without* and a one represents *with.* In six-character codes, a one represents *with* and a nine represents *without.*

The phrase *other specified* is included in some code titles and means that the information in the health record provides detail for which a specific code is not provided in the classification. Conversely, the word *unspecified* in a code title indicates that the information in the health record is not sufficient to support a more specific code.

Two phrases connote special meaning in the ICD-10-CM Tabular List: *not elsewhere classified* (or *classifiable*) and *not otherwise specified.* The inclusion of *not elsewhere classified* in a category or code title indicates that there may be another code that provides greater specificity for the condition to be coded. It should be considered an indicator that a better code is not available. For example, code J15, Bacterial pneumonia, not elsewhere classified, should be assigned only when it has been determined that the condition being coded cannot be reported by using a more specific code in some other category in the classification system.

When *not otherwise specified* appears in the Tabular List, users should recognize that the code is to be assigned only when no additional information about the condition has been documented. For example:

A06.0 Acute amebic dysentery
Acute amebiasis
Intestinal amebiasis NOS

A06.0 should be used only when the intestinal amebiasis is not qualified or modified in any other way.

In the following example, the **includes** statement indicates that infectious colitis that is not otherwise specified or further described is included in category A09. Similarly, the **excludes** statement indicates that colitis, diarrhea, and so on, which are not otherwise specified or modified, are not included in the category.

A09   Infectious gastroenteritis and colitis, unspecified
    Includes: infectious colitis NOS
                     infectious enteritis NOS
                     infectious gastroenteritis NOS
    Excludes 1:   colitis NOS (K52.9)
                     diarrhea NOS (R19.7)
                     enteritis NOS (K52.9)
                     gastroenteritis NOS (K52.9)
                     noninfective gastroenteritis and colitis, unspecified (K52.9)

Notes

Includes and *excludes* notes are also used as conventions in the ICD-10-CM Tabular List. ICD-10-CM uses inclusion terms and *includes* notes to clarify which conditions are included in a particular category. The inclusion terms serve as examples of the diagnostic statements that are included in a particular category. For example:

A39.1   Waterhouse–Friderichsen syndrome
       Meningococcal hemorrhagic adrenalitis
       Meningoccocic adrenal syndrome

K45   Other abdominal hernia
    Includes: abdominal hernia, specified site
                   lumbar hernia
                   obturator hernia
                   pudendal hernia
                   retroperitoneal hernia
                   sciatic hernia

In some instances, the word *includes* does not precede the list of terms included in the code. For example:

K52.9   Noninfective gastroenteritis and colitis, unspecified
       Colitis NOS
       Enteritis NOS
       Gastroenteritis NOS
       Ileitis NOS
       Jejunitis NOS
       Sigmoiditis NOS

It is important to note that lists of inclusion terms are not exhaustive and may include diagnoses not listed as inclusion terms. The Alphabetic Index of ICD-10-CM may direct the users to assign a particular code even though it is not listed as an inclusion term.

Includes notes may appear under a chapter or block title to provide general information about the content of the chapter or block. For example:

P07   Disorders of newborn related to short gestation and low birth weight, not elsewhere classified
    Note: When both birth weight and gestational age of the newborn are available, both should be coded, with birth weight sequenced before gestational age.
    Includes: the listed conditions, without further specification, as the cause of morbidity or additional care, in newborn

Many categories and subcategories contain a list of conditions preceded by the word *excludes*. **Excludes** notes indicate that the conditions listed should be classified to some other category or subcategory. They should be read very carefully because they often indicate the category or subcategory to which the excluded term should be assigned. For example:

K60   Fissure and fistula of anal and rectal regions
     Excludes 1:   fissure and fistula of anal and rectal regions with abscess or cellulitis (K61.–)
    K60.4   Rectal fistula
       Fistula of rectum to skin
       Excludes 1:   rectovaginal fistula (N82.3)
                   vesicorectal fistula (N32.1)

In some cases, the Tabular List will not direct the user to another category or subcategory but, rather, to the Alphabetic Index. For example:

Z39.0   Encounter for care and examination of mother immediately after delivery
     Care and observation in uncomplicated cases when the delivery occurs outside a healthcare facility
     Excludes 1:   care for postpartum complications—see Alphabetic Index

ICD-10-CM provides two types of **excludes** notes, each of which is identified by the number one or two:

- **Excludes 1** notes designate codes that can never be used together because the two conditions represented by the codes would never occur together. This type of **excludes** note is easy to apply.

- **Excludes 2** notes indicate that the excluded condition is a separate condition that is not a part of, or included in, the condition represented by the code. In some instances, these notes mean that using more than one code to completely represent the patient's illness would be appropriate.

Examples of **excludes** notes include:

F31   Bipolar disorder
    Includes: manic-depressive illness
                  manic-depressive psychosis
                  manic-depressive reaction
    Excludes 1:   bipolar disorder, single manic episode (F30.–)
                  major depressive disorder, single episode (F32.–)
                  major depressive disorder, recurrent (F33.–)
    Excludes 2:   cyclothymia (F34.0)

D72   Other disorders of white blood cells
    Excludes 1:   basophilia (D75.8)
                  immunity disorders (D80–D89)
                  netropenia (D70)
                  preleukemia (syndrome) (D46.9)

K44   Diaphragmatic hernia
    Includes: paraesophageal hernia
                    hiatus hernia (esophageal) (sliding)
    Excludes 1:   congenital diaphragmatic hernia (Q79.0)
                    congenital hiatus hernia (Q40.1)

Q83   Congenital malformations of breast
    Excludes 2:   absence of pectoral muscle (Q79.8)

Code first/use additional code notes identify codes that describe both the cause (etiology) and the subsequent manifestation of a condition and remind the user that one code may be more appropriate to use than separate codes that identify the etiology and the manifestation. For example:

B39   Histoplasmosis
    Code first associated AIDS (B20)
    Use additional code for any associated manifestations, such as:
        endocarditis (I39)
        meningitis (G02)
        pericarditis (I32)
        retinitis (H32)

J15   Bacterial pneumonia, not elsewhere classified
    Code first any associated lung abscess (J85.1)

The *use additional code* note is similar to the *code first* note in that the *use additional code* note indicates that an additional code may be needed to completely describe a condition. Many of the notes warn users to assign an additional code to identify the external cause of a condition (for example, dermatitis), an associated condition (for example, Crohn's disease with pyoderma gangrenosum), or the nature of the condition (for example, the type of infection). When two codes are appropriate, the manifestation code should be sequenced first before the etiology code.

Depending on the situation, these notes may give specific codes or a range of codes. The phrase *such as* should be interpreted to mean *for example* and to indicate that the list is not exhaustive but simply provides several common examples. Additional examples include:

I30.1   Infective pericarditis
    Use additional code (B95–B97) to identify infectious agent

J17   Pneumonia in diseases classified elsewhere
    Code first underlying disease, such as:
        Q fever (A78)
        rheumatic fever (I00)
        schistosomiasis (B65.0–B65.9)
        septicemia (A40.0-A41.9)
    Code first any associated lung abscess (J85.1)
    Excludes 1:   candidial pneumonia (B37.1)
                  chlamydial pneumonia (J16.0)
                  gonorrheal pneumonia (A54.84)
                  histoplasmosis pneumonia (B39.0–B39.2)

J68   Respiratory conditions due to inhalation of chemicals, gases, fumes and vapors
    Code first (T51–T65) to identify cause

Terminology

The word *and* should be interpreted to mean *and/or* in the Tabular List. For example, in code A18.4, Tuberculosis of skin and subcutaneous tissue, tuberculosis of the skin or tuberculosis of the subcutaneous tissue or tuberculosis of the skin and subcutaneous tissue would all be included.

The word *with* is used to refer to combinations of conditions. For example, for code K21.0, Gastro-esophageal reflux disease with esophagitis, both the reflux disease and the esophagitis must be present.

Other Conventions Followed in the Tabular List

During the process of modifying ICD-10 to create ICD-10-CM, some ICD-10 codes were deemed inactive and cannot be reassigned under the ICD-10-CM classification. For example, a note appears just before the beginning of the T codes that indicates that categories T00 through T06 are deactivated and that the individual injuries should be coded.

ICD-10-CM uses lowercase exes in codes to act as placeholders so that additional detail could be included in the classification system in the future. For example:

T36.0x	Poisoning by, adverse effect of and underdosing of penicillins
T36.0x1	Poisoning by penicillins, accidental (unintentional)
T36.0x2	Poisoning by penicillins, intentional self-harm
T36.0x3	Poisoning by penicillins, assault
T36.0x4	Poisoning by penicillins, undetermined
T36.0x5	Adverse effect of penicillins
T36.0x6	Underdosing of penicillins

The ICD-9-CM conventions that used braces to enclose a series of terms and section mark symbols to denote the placement of footnotes have not been employed in ICD-10-CM.

Alphabetic Index

The Alphabetic Index for ICD-10-CM can be roughly divided into three sections:

- The first section is the index to the terms classifiable to chapters 1 through 19 and 21, except drugs and chemicals. This section includes the Table of Neoplasms.

- The second section is the index to the terms related to the external causes of morbidity and terms classifiable to chapter 20.

- The third section is the Table of Drugs and Chemicals, which is used to code poisonings and adverse effects of drugs classifiable to chapters 19 and 20.

The Alphabetic Index is organized by main terms set in boldface type. The main terms generally identify conditions rather than anatomic structures. For example, to find the correct code for irritable colon, the users should refer to the main term *irritable* rather than *colon*.

Many entries are not strictly disease conditions, however. Codes from chapter 21, Factors influencing health status and contact with health services, are found under main terms such as Admission (for), Aftercare, Boarder, Convalescence, Examination, History, Prescription, Problem, State of, Status, and Vaccination.

Modifiers are also known as qualifiers. Subterms, or essential modifiers, are located under main terms at various indentation levels. Nonessential modifiers appear in parentheses and do not affect the code number assigned. Subterms may be modified by other modifiers. A typical Alphabetic Index entry looks like the following:

Adenocarcinoma-in-situ
(M8140/2)—see also
Neoplasm, in situ
-breast (female)   D05.90
--male   D05.95
-in
--adenoma (polypoid)
(tubular) (M8210/0)
---tubulovillous (M8263/2)
---villous (M8261/2)
---polyp, adenomatous
(M8210/2)

In the index of terms related to external causes, main terms and modifiers indicate types of accidents or occurrences, vehicles involved, places of occurrence, and so on. For example:

Accident (to)   X58.8
-aircraft (in transit) (powered)
--see also Accident,
transport, aircraft due to, caused by
cataclysm—see Forces of nature, by type
-animal-rider—see Accident, transport,
animal-rider
-animal-drawn vehicle—see Accident,
transport, animal-drawn
vehicle occupant
-automobile—see Accident, transport,
car occupant
-bare foot water skier   V94.4
-boat, boating—see also Accident, watercraft
striking swimmer
--powered   V94.11
--unpowered   V94.12
-bus—see Accident, transport, bus occupant
-cable car, not on rails   V98.0
--on rails—see Accident, transport,
streetcar occupant

Conventions Followed in the Alphabetic Index

Two additional conventions are followed in the Alphabetic Index: the use of the abbreviation NEC and the use of cross-reference terms.

Abbreviation: NEC

The abbreviation NEC (not elsewhere classified) is used in the Alphabetic Index to flag general terms. NEC serves to remind the users to look for a more specific code. For example:

17

Observation (for) (without
need for further medical care)
Z04.9
-accident NEC   Z04.3
--at work   Z04.2
--transport   Z04.1
.
.
.
-suicide attempt, alleged
NEC   Z03.8
--self-poisoning   Z03.6

In the preceding example, code Z03.8 would be used for an attempted suicide, but the user should determine whether a more specific code—such as Z03.6, Suicide attempt by self-poisoning—would be more appropriate. The general code Z04.3 also can be used to indicate an accident, not elsewhere classified, although codes Z04.2 and Z04.1 are more specific.

Cross-Reference Terms

Several types of cross-reference devices are used in the Alphabetic Index to make identifying the correct codes easier. For example, a *see* cross-reference directs users to another main term. For example:

Glass-blower's disease (cataract)—see Cataract, specified NEC

Iselin's disease or osteochondrosis—see Osteochondrosis, juvenile, metatarsus

Chest—see condition

See also cross-references direct the user to another main term when the information under the first main term is not sufficient to assign an accurate code. For example:

Onyxitis—see also Cellulitis, digit

Cystadenocarcinoma (M8440/3)—see also Neoplasm, malignant

Cross-references occasionally direct users to *see* or *see also* another category or code in the Tabular List rather than to refer to another term in the Alphabetic Index. For example:

Isoimmunization NEC—see also
Incompatibility
-affecting management of
pregnancy (ABO)—see also
subcategory   O36.1
Maternal care (for)
-see Pregnancy
(complicated by)
(management affected by)

Table of Neoplasms

The Table of Neoplasms in the Alphabetic Index is arranged in alphabetic order by anatomic site. For each site listed, six code numbers are possible, depending on whether the neoplasm is malignant (primary or secondary), benign, in situ, of uncertain behavior, or of unspecified behavior.

Implementation and Training Issues

Implementation of ICD-10-CM in the United States will present a number of challenges. Several organizations have recommended that the Department of Health and Human Services issue a proposal requiring U.S. healthcare facilities to adopt the ICD-10-CM code set as the national standard. Adoption of ICD-10-CM as the national code set, however, presents numerous issues in terms of training personnel to use the code set and adapting current information systems. Canada and Australia have both modified ICD-10 for use in their countries, and their training efforts and methodologies provide models that the United States can study in determining its implementation strategies.

Code Sets

In August 2000, the Department of Health and Human Services released the final rule for transaction and medical code sets as established under the Health Insurance Portability and Accountability Act. To be designated as a HIPPA standard, a code set had to:

- Improve the efficiency and effectiveness of the healthcare system by leading to cost reductions for or improvement in benefits from electronic healthcare transactions

- Meet the needs of the health data standards user community, particularly healthcare providers, health plans, and healthcare clearinghouses

- Be consistent and uniform with other HIPAA standards—their data element definitions and codes and privacy and security requirements—and, secondarily, with other private and public sector health data standards

- Have low additional development and implementation costs relative to the benefits of using the standard

- Be supported by an ANSI-accredited standards development organization or other private or public organization that would ensure continuity and efficient updating of the standard over time

- Have timely development, testing, implementation, and updating procedures to achieve administrative simplification benefits faster

- Be technologically independent of the computer platforms and transmission protocols used in electronic health transactions, except when they are explicitly part of the standard

- Be precise and unambiguous but as simple as possible

- Keep data collection and paperwork burdens on users as low as is feasible

- Incorporate flexibility to adapt more easily to changes in the healthcare infrastructure, such as new services, organizations, and provider types and information technology (*Federal Register* 1998)

This final rule designated five medical code sets to be used for assigning diagnoses and procedures. These are:

- *International Classification of Diseases, Ninth Revision, Clinical Modification* (ICD-9-CM)

- *Current Procedural Terminology, Fourth Edition* (CPT-4)

- *Healthcare Common Procedural Coding System* (HCPCS)

- *Code on Dental Procedures and Nomenclature, Second Edition* (CDT-2)

- *National Drug Codes* (NDC)

(The mandated use of NCD codes for use in nonretail pharmacy transactions was repealed by the HHS in 2003.)

The final rule became effective on October 16, 2000. Most entities were required to comply by October 16, 2002, although many organizations received an extension and had until October 16, 2003, to become compliant.

ICD-10-CM Proposed as a National Code Set

Various organizations have recommended that the HHS issue a proposed rule requiring that facilities adopt the new ICD-10-CM codes as the national standard code set. Among these organizations are the American Health Information Management Association (AHIMA), the American Academy of Professional Coders, the American Hospital Association (AHA), the Advanced Medical Technology Association, the American Medical Association (AMA), and the Federation of American Hospitals (Prophet 2002). In a letter dated November 19, 2002, members of the AHA, the Advanced Medical Technology Association, and the Federation of American Hospitals indicated that "the 23-year-old ICD-9-CM coding classification system has severely limited reporting capabilities for today's needs and no growth capacity for future needs, making it an increasingly unacceptable coding classification system for the future for both inpatient and outpatient diagnosis, as well as hospital inpatient services' procedure coding" (AHA et al. 2002).

The AHIMA believes that ICD-10-CM represents a "significant improvement over both ICD-9-CM and ICD-10" (Prophet 2002). Furthermore, the AHIMA contends that ICD-9-CM is outdated and obsolete and that adoption of ICD-10-CM is an absolute necessity. Even the HHS noted that ICD-9-CM did not meet all of the HIPAA requirements for adopted standards, citing ambiguity, lack of precision, and lack of desired level of flexibility (*Federal Register* 1998).

In testimony before the Subcommittee on Standards and Security of the National Committee on Vital and Health Statistics on May 29, 2002, Sue Prophet, director of coding policy and compliance for the AHIMA, indicated that "the level of specificity in ICD-10-CM will provide payers, policy makers, and providers with more detailed information for establishing appropriate reimbursement rates, evaluating and improving quality of patient care, improving efficiencies in healthcare delivery, reducing healthcare costs, and effectively monitoring resource and service utilization" (Prophet 2002).

Principles for Code Set Maintenance

Code set maintenance is another challenge that will need to be met after the implementation of ICD-10-CM. The AHIMA has developed the following recommendations and principles for code set maintenance (Prophet 2002, attachment #3):

1. The committee responsible for system maintenance should be composed of representatives from all major stakeholder groups, including the government, healthcare providers, and private payers.

2. The maintenance process should be open, with public meetings (broadcast live over the Internet) and opportunities for public input both at and outside formal meetings.

3. Due to rapid advances in medicine and technology and the immediate need for codes to describe such advances, the maintenance process should be more streamlined, with consideration given to the feasibility of more frequent system updates.

4. The lag time between the proposal of a new code and its implementation should be minimized.

5. A process should be established for developing rules and guidelines for the correct application of the coding system. The process should be open and permit broad input from all stakeholders prior to finalization of a significantly revised or changed guideline. The coding system rules and guidelines (and consequent payment system changes) should be updated on the same schedule as the code set and made part of the official version.

6. All requisite materials—code sets, guidelines, and other directives—should be in formats available from government or private entities. This would ensure that all stakeholders know where to go for unfettered access to the official, most up-to-date versions, and interpretive materials.

ICD-10-CM Training Issues

Before discussing ICD-10-CM implementation in the United States, a review of the adoption process that has taken place in other countries is appropriate. The AHIMA surveyed several other countries regarding their implementation strategies and the obstacles they encountered. Interestingly, the AHIMA discovered that many other countries are disgruntled about the failure of the United States to adopt ICD-10 and about the resulting unavailability of comparable worldwide data.

As mentioned previously, both Australia and Canada have developed modifications of ICD-10 for use in their countries. ICD-10-AM and ICD-10-CA were developed with the permission of the WHO, as was ICD-10-CM. ICD-10-AM has been fully implemented in Australia since 1999, and most of Canada has completed the conversion to ICD-10-CA. In both countries, implementation was phased in over the course of two years. Canada has an entirely electronic ICD-10-CA product; no printed ICD-10-CA code books are available. Australia and Canada adopted ICD-10 because of the need for a more clinically useful case-mix index and also because of its applicability in non-acute care settings.

In Australia, the National Center for Classification in Health (NCCH) formed an ICD-10-AM Education Working Party composed of individuals from educational facilities, professional organizations, and NCCH Education Division staff. Between 1995 and 1999, the NCCH conducted training courses and developed educational materials. In addition, postimplementation workshops were held to clarify coding issues.

The NCCH prepared and distributed ICD-10-AM implementation kits to all healthcare facilities. These kits included information briefing (fact) sheets and visual aids on topics such as the background behind the move to ICD-10-AM, details about the classification system, stages of the implementation process, and information on transitional issues. In addition, the NCCH released six booklets on various topics related to implementing the new system. Finally, the NCCH released the *Mastering Ten* exercise workbook, which was a self-instructional tool (Innes, Peasley, and Roberts 2000).

Canada provided coding education in a three-phase plan. The first phase consisted of a self-learning package that required about twenty-one hours to complete. The second phase consisted of a two-day workshop, with a hands-on program. In the third phase, a self-learning package of ten case studies was provided to users. All of the education in Canada involved the use of coding software and not code books. Both countries offer periodic refresher courses. The average learning curve was four to six months, and users reported that they did not find ICD-10 any more or less difficult to learn than ICD-9 (Prophet 2002).

Just as was done in Australia, the first step to make in planning an implementation strategy for an individual facility in the United States should be to create a committee, team, or task force to oversee the implementation process. Certainly, upper management should be represented as well as all departments affected in any way by the change. At the very least, the task force should include representatives from the health information management (HIM) department, information systems or services, the billing department, the accounting department, human/personnel resources, and the medical staff. The frequency of meetings should depend on the individual facility and the responsibilities of the task force.

One of the first questions to address is, Who will be affected by the change to ICD-10-CM? Many more individuals are affected today because the uses of coded data have changed so much since adoption of ICD-9-CM more than 23 years ago. Obviously, coding professionals and physicians will require training, but other individuals also will be affected and thus will need some training depending on the extent of their involvement.

Educational efforts may take many forms. Face-to-face workshops or seminars will continue to be an important part of any type of retraining program, but there are several alternatives for individuals who cannot travel to a seminar or workshop. Currently, a number of excellent coding publications are dedicated to coding training. It is expected that similar tools will be published for ICD-10-CM. Audio seminars that deliver information to a large audience are cost-effective because no travel is involved. Certainly, Web-based training will play an important role. Many vendors already have excellent coding programs available that presumably will be adapted to ICD-10-CM. Web-based training is particularly effective in training large numbers of individuals and can be highly effective, depending on the quality of the program and the dedication of the participants.

Various methodologies should be employed because people learn new information in a variety of ways. For instance, physicians may respond better to face-to-face presentations than to Web-based training programs.

Educators in coding certificate programs, health information technology programs, and health information administration programs will be charged with the task of training new coding professionals. Training materials will take advantage of information technology, and ensuring the availability of computers may prove to be a challenge for some educational facilities. Students enrolled in HIM programs will need to be trained in both the ICD-9-CM and ICD-10-CM classification systems even after ICD-10-CM has been implemented so that they will be able to manage ICD-9-CM-based historical data.

Training for Coding Professionals

Although ICD-10-CM is different from ICD-9-CM in many ways, the new classification system retains the traditional format and many of the same characteristics and conventions. Thus, experienced coding professionals should have little difficulty in achieving coding proficiency. Experienced coding professionals will require education on changes in the structure of the codes, definitions, and guidelines. There are many more trained coding professionals today than there were when ICD-9-CM was introduced, but less-experienced users will face a number of challenges. The increased level of specificity with ICD-10-CM will require a strong foundation in anatomy and physiology, medical terminology, pharmacology, and medical science.

An additional problem that could be encountered is a shortage of credentialed coding professionals. Currently, there is a shortage of coding professionals skilled in both ICD-9-CM and CPT coding, and some experienced professionals may opt to retire rather than to learn a new system. Labor statistics predict a continued shortage of qualified coding professionals in the near future.

Training for Physicians

The inadequacy of physician documentation has been an obstacle to complete and accurate coding for some time. With the increased specificity in ICD-10-CM, this problem will continue to be a factor in the collection of accurate statistical data as well as the key to appropriate reimbursement. The level of specificity required in ICD-10-CM demands that physicians be educated to meet the information requirements of the new system. A careful review of the code changes for ICD-10-CM clearly demonstrates the necessity of complete documentation and the use of current terminology. Having physicians actively involved in the implementation process allows them the opportunity to understand the importance of complete and accurate health record documentation.

In addition to the training methods previously discussed, documentation assessment will continue to be an important tool for improving physician documentation. Results of the assessments can be shared with the physicians, and instances where patient care was compromised or revenue was lost because of inadequate documentation can be highlighted. Information on the uses of coded data apart from reimbursement should be shared with physicians as well so that they can better understand the impact of documentation.

Training for Other Healthcare Professionals

The many users of health record data will require varying levels of training, depending on their involvement with coded data. Some of these users include:

- Clinicians other than physicians such as nurses and allied health professionals

- Quality management personnel

- Utilization management and case management personnel

- Data quality and data security personnel

- Researchers, data analysts, and epidemiologists

- Software vendors

- Information systems personnel

- Billing, decision support, and accounting personnel

- Compliance officers

- Internal and external auditors and consulting firms

- Fraud investigators

- Government agency personnel

Certainly, all healthcare professionals who provide patient care should receive training in ICD-10-CM. Training techniques similar to those outlined for physicians can be used.

Because ICD-10-CM will require concise and specific documentation from physicians and other clinical practitioners, the implementation of ICD-10-CM will benefit researchers and data analysts. Better data will "improve the ability of providers, payers, the government and others to measure the quality, safety and efficacy of care; support providers' and payers' performance improvement activities; improve public health surveillance; and enhance health policy decision-making" (Prophet 2002). Some data analysts are already using ICD-10. For example, data analysts who work with international data are familiar with the system.

One of the significant challenges posed by implementing ICD-10-CM is the readiness of the software vendors. Experiences in both Australia and Canada have shown that vendors were not prepared for the change despite the planning time available. With sufficient preparation time, U.S. vendors should have software available in a timely fashion. Many facilities may use electronic versions rather than printed codebooks because of the length of the new classification.

Impact on Information Systems

The move to ICD-10-CM might be compared to Y2K in the amount of work faced by information systems personnel. All electronic transactions requiring a diagnosis and/or procedure code will need to be reviewed (and possibly changed). Some of the various systems that will need to reviewed include: billing systems, decision support systems, clinical systems, encoding software, health record abstracting systems, aggregate data reporting, utilization and quality management systems, case-mix systems, accounting systems, clinical protocols, test-ordering systems, clinical reminder systems, performance measurement systems, medical necessity software, and benefits determination (Prophet 2002; Ingenix 2002).

Software will need to be developed to accommodate field size expansion, alphanumeric codes, redefinitions of code values, edit and logic changes, modifications of table structure, and expansion of flat files containing diagnosis codes and systems interfaces (Prophet 2002). Some specific examples include:

- Any field that requires a code will need to accommodate up to seven characters rather than five.

- Any field that requires a code will need to be changed to accept alphanumeric codes rather in addition to numeric codes. (This may not be an issue because of the V codes and E codes already used in ICD-9-CM.)

- Some reprogramming may be needed to differentiate between letters and numbers that tend to be hard to distinguish (for example, the number one and the lowercase letter el).

- ICD-10-CM codes may have up to four characters (numbers or letters) after the decimal point. In ICD-9-CM, there is a maximum of only two numbers after the decimal point.

- The size of data fields accommodating descriptions of the codes may have to be reviewed. Code titles are much more descriptive and thus longer in ICD-10-CM than in ICD-9-CM.

- ICD-10-CM offers many more codes than ICD-9-CM does. Therefore, the hardware will need to be able to accommodate additional data. Both ICD-9-CM and ICD-10-CM will have to be supported by the computer hardware.

- ICD-10-CM codes that consist of five characters may be confused with HCPCS Level II codes, which also begin with an alphabetic character. This will not be a problem if the decimal point is placed in the ICD-10-CM codes, but it might be a problem if the software did not use the decimal.

Impact on Reimbursement

Several training issues need to be addressed with billing and accounting personnel. First, the chief financial officer (CFO) of the organization will need to look at capital expenditures such as new or upgraded hardware, new software, training costs for coding professionals and other personnel, and, finally, the hiring of information systems personnel to accomplish the changeover.

In addition, there will likely be delays in payments from third-party payers until coders and billing personnel are fully trained on the system. Moreover, there may be increased numbers of claims denials or rejections due to inadequate coding, reporting, and processing.

Initially, payments should not be substantially affected from the standpoint of reimbursement systems. It is expected that ICD-10-CM codes will be mapped to ICD-9-CM codes and that ICD-9-CM data will continue to be used in assigning reimbursement rates until sufficient ICD-10-CM data are available. At some point, managed care contracts and negotiated rate schedules will be recalculated using ICD-10-CM data.

Eventually, ICD-10-CM data will "allow appropriate refinements of reimbursement systems to better reflect the actual cost of patient care; will improve providers' and payers' ability to negotiate reimbursement rates; improve payers' ability to forecast the healthcare needs and analyze healthcare costs; reduce payers' and providers' costs due to improved ability to effectively monitor service and resource utilization, analyze healthcare costs, monitor outcomes, measure performance, and detect fraud and abuse" (Prophet 2002). Moreover, the increased specificity should reduce the number of requests for medical records to justify payment because the codes should provide the information needed.

Impact on Human Resources

Even human resource managers will be affected by the changeover to ICD-10-CM. With the adoption of the new system, qualified coding professionals will be in demand, and retention of trained coding professionals will be essential to the facility's billing function. Thus, facilities may need to reevaluate salary structures and benefit packages to ensure that they are competitive with other institutions.

References

American Hospital Association, Advanced Medical Technology Association, and the Federation of American Hospitals. 2002. November 20, 2002, letter to members of the National Committee on Vital and Health Statistics. Available from www.healthdatamanagement.com/HDMSearchResultsDetails.cfm?DID=13512.

Federal Register. May 7, 1998. (Volume 63, number 8, pp. 25272–25320.) Available from www.access.gpo/su_docs/aces/aces140.

Ingenix. 2002. *Ingenix Coding Lab: Implementing ICD-10.* Reston, Va.: Ingenix.

Innes, Kerry, Karen Peasley, and Rosemary Roberts. 2000. Ten down under: implementing ICD-10 in Australia. *Journal of the American Health Information Management Association* 71(1):52–56.

National Center for Health Statistics. 2003. Official coding guidelines for ICD-10-CM. Available at www.cdc.gov/nchs/about/otheract/icd9/abticd10.htm.

Prophet, Sue. 2002. Testimony before members of the National Committee on Vital and Health Statistics (NCVHS), Standards and Security Subcommittee, May 29, 2002. Available from www.ahima.org/dc/comments.ncvhs.052902.cfm.

Chapter 1

Infectious and Parasitic Diseases

Chapter 1 in the ICD-10-CM Tabular List is entitled Certain infectious and parasitic diseases. It includes categories A00 through B99 and is arranged in the following blocks:

A00–A09	Intestinal infectious diseases
A15–A19	Tuberculosis
A20–A28	Certain zoonotic bacterial diseases
A30–A49	Other bacterial diseases
A50–A64	Infections with a predominantly sexual mode of transmission
A65–A69	Other spirochetal diseases
A70–A74	Other diseases caused by chlamydiae
A75–A79	Rickettsioses
A80–A89	Viral infections of the central nervous system
A90–A99	Arthropod-borne viral fevers and viral hemorrhagic fevers
B00–B09	Viral infections characterized by skin and mucous membrane lesions
B15–B19	Viral hepatitis
B20	Human immunodeficiency virus [HIV] disease
B25–B34	Other viral diseases
B35–B49	Mycoses
B50–B64	Protozoal diseases
B65–B83	Helminthiases
B85–B89	Pediculosis, acariasis and other infestations
B90–B94	Sequelae of infectious and parasitic diseases
B95–B97	Bacterial, viral and other infectious agents
B99	Other infectious diseases

Title Changes

A number of block, category, and subcategory title changes have been made in chapter 1 of ICD-10-CM. A few examples of these changes include:

ICD-9-CM:	Zoonotic Bacterial Diseases (020–027)	
ICD-10-CM:	Certain zoonotic bacterial diseases (A20–A28)	
ICD-9-CM:	Late Effects of Infectious and Parasitic Diseases (137–139)	
ICD-10-CM:	Sequelae of infectious and parasitic diseases (B90–B94)	
ICD-9-CM:	006.6	Amebic skin ulceration
ICD-10-CM:	A06.7	Cutaneous amebiasis
ICD-9-CM:	005	Other food poisoning (bacterial)
ICD-10-CM:	A05	Other bacterial foodborne intoxications
ICD-9-CM:	121	Other trematode infections
ICD-10-CM:	B66	Other fluke infections

Additions, Deletions, and Combinations

When chapter 1 in ICD-10-CM is compared with chapter 1 in ICD-9-CM, it is evident that many codes have been added, deleted, combined, or moved to another section or chapter. For example, several codes were moved from one section to another. These types of changes should not present a problem for coding professionals because the Alphabetic Index provides directions to the correct codes. For example:

- Cat-scratch fever was moved from Diseases due to viral agents (078.3) to Zoonotic bacterial disease (A28.1).

- Leptospirosis (100) was moved from Spirochetal disease to Certain zoonotic bacterial diseases (A20–A28).

Other codes have been moved from one chapter to another. For example, the code for tetanus neonatorum has been moved from chapter 15, Certain Conditions Originating in the Perinatal Period (760–779), in ICD-9-CM to chapter 1 in ICD-10-CM and is coded to A33, Tetanus neonatorum. Also, obstetrical tetanus has been moved from category 670 in the obstetrics chapter of ICD-9-CM to category A34 in chapter 1 of ICD-10-CM.

Chapter 1 of ICD-10-CM includes a new section called Infections with a predominantly sexual mode of transmission (A50–A64). Many codes have been moved into this section from other places in the ICD-9-CM classification. An exception is HIV disease, which is excluded from this section and classified to B20.

Included in this section are the codes for syphilis, which have been expanded. For example:

ICD-9-CM:	091.3	Secondary syphilis of skin or mucous membranes
ICD-10-CM:	A51.3	Secondary syphilis of skin and mucous membranes
	A51.31	Condyloma latum
	A51.32	Syphilitic alopecia
	A51.39	Other secondary syphilis of skin

Codes for gonococcal infection (A54), which also fall into this block, are no longer classified according to whether the condition is acute or chronic. The axis for the fourth-character subcategory is the site of the gonococcal infection. For example:

ICD-9-CM:	098.0	Gonococcal infection, acute, of lower genitourinary tract
ICD-10-CM:	A54.0	Gonococcal infection of lower genitourinary tract without periurethral or accessory gland abscess

Some conditions have been assigned new category codes in ICD-10-CM. For example:

ICD-9-CM: 099   Other venereal diseases
             099.0   Chancroid
             099.1   Lymphogranuloma venereum
             099.2   Granuloma inguinale
ICD-10-CM: A57   Chancroid
             A58   Granuloma inguinale

Expansions

A number of codes for infectious and parasitic diseases have been expanded in ICD-10-CM.

Typhoid Fever

The code for typhoid fever (A01.0) has been expanded in ICD-10-CM to reflect the manifestations of typhoid fever. For example:

ICD-9-CM: 002.0   Typhoid fever
ICD-10-CM: A01.0   Typhoid fever
                     Infection due to Salmonella typhi
             A01.00 Typhoid fever, unspecified
             A01.01 Typhoid meningitis
             A01.02 Typhoid fever with heart involvement
             A01.03 Typhoid pneumonia
             A01.04 Typhoid arthritis
             A01.05 Typhoid osteomyelitis
             A01.09 Typhoid fever with other complications

Amebic Infections

The code for amebic infection of other sites (A06.8) has been expanded to fifth characters to indicate specific sites. For example:

ICD-9-CM: 006.8   Amebic infection of other sites
ICD-10-CM: A06.8   Amebic infection of other sites
             A06.81 Amebic cystitis
             A06.82 Other amebic genitourinary infections
             A06.89 Other amebic infections

Intestinal Infections

ICD-9-CM category 008, Intestinal infections due to other organisms, has been split into three category codes in ICD-10-CM: A04, Other bacterial intestinal infections; A08, Viral and other specified intestinal infections; and A09, Infectious gastroenteritis and colitis, unspecified.

Tuberculosis

The tuberculosis codes have been restructured with consolidation of some categories. For example, ICD-9-CM category codes 011, Pulmonary tuberculosis, and 012, Other respiratory tuberculosis, have been consolidated into A15, Respiratory tuberculosis. Similarly, ICD-9-CM category codes 013, Tuberculosis of meninges and central nervous system; 014, Tuberculosis of intestines, peritoneum and mesenteric glands; 015, Tuberculosis of bones and joints; 016, Tuberculosis of genitourinary system; and 017, Tuberculosis of other organs, have been combined into categories A17, Tuberculosis of nervous system, and A18, Tuberculosis of other organs. There is no code comparable to 010, Primary tuberculosis, in ICD-10-CM. In addition, rubric A16 is not used in ICD-10-CM.

Expansions to Category Codes

In numerous instances, codes included as subcategory codes in ICD-9-CM are given a specific category code in ICD-10-CM and expanded at the fourth- or fifth-character level. For example:

ICD-9-CM: 027.1   Erysipelothrix infection
ICD-10-CM: A26   Erysipeloid
           A26.0   Cutaneous erysipeloid
           A26.7   Erysipelothrix septicemia
           A26.8   Other forms of erysipeloid
           A26.9   Erysipeloid, unspecified

ICD-9-CM: 116.0   Blastomycosis
ICD-10-CM: B40   Blastomycosis
           B40.0   Acute pulmonary blastomycosis
           B40.1   Chronic pulmonary blastomycosis
           B40.2   Pulmonary blastomycosis, unspecified
           B40.3   Cutaneous blastomycosis
           B40.7   Disseminated blastomycosis
           B40.8   Other forms of blastomycosis
                 B40.81   Blastomycotic meningoencephalitis
                 B40.89   Other forms of blastomycosis
           B40.9   Blastomycosis, unspecified

ICD-9-CM: 116.1   Paracoccidioidomycosis
ICD-10-CM: B41   Paracoccidioidomycosis
           B41.0   Pulmonary paracoccidioidomycosis
           B41.7   Disseminated paracoccidioidomycosis
           B41.8   Other forms of paracoccidioidomycosis
           B41.9   Paracoccidioidomycosis, unspecified

Other categories that have been expanded include B42, Sporotrichosis; B44, Aspergillosis; B45, Cryptococcosis; B46, Zygomycosis; and B69, Cysticercosis. Changes in these categories should be conveyed to physicians to make them aware of the documentation needed for accurate coding.

Expansions to Include Manifestations

Many of the codes in chapter 1 of ICD-10-CM have been expanded to reflect manifestations of the disease with the use of fourth or fifth characters, rather than the use of an additional code, to identify the manifestation. Some examples include:

ICD-9-CM: 027.0   Listeriosis
                        Use additional code to identify manifestation, as meningitis (320.7)

ICD-10-CM: A32   Listeriosis
                    A32.0   Cutaneous listeriosis
                    A32.1   Listerial meningitis and meningoencephalitis
                            A32.11   Listerial meningitis
                            A32.12   Listerial meningoencephalitis
                    A32.7   Listerial sepsis
                    A32.8   Other forms of listeriosis
                            A32.81   Oculoglandular listeriosis
                            A32.82   Listerial endocarditis
                            A32.89   Other forms of listeriosis
                    A32.9   Listeriosis, unspecified

ICD-9-CM: 033   Whooping cough
                        Use additional code to identify any associated pneumonia (484.3)

ICD-10-CM: A37   Whooping cough
                    A37.0   Whooping cough due to Bordetella pertussis
                            A37.00   Whooping cough due to Bordetella pertussis without pneumonia
                            A37.01   Whooping cough due to Bordetella pertussis with pneumonia

In some instances, opposite changes have been made. For example, in ICD-9-CM, fifth digits reflect manifestations, but in ICD-10-CM, a note directs the user to "use additional code for any associated manifestation." For example, in ICD-9-CM, category 115, Histoplasmosis, has fifth digits that reflect any manifestations of the disease. In ICD-10-CM, category B39, Histoplasmosis, includes a note directing the coder to use an additional code for the associated manifestation, such as endocarditis or pericarditis.

Sepsis

Septicemia (ICD-9-CM category 038) is assigned two category codes in ICD-10-CM: A40, Streptococcal sepsis, and A41, Other sepsis. Both of these category codes have instructions to code first certain conditions. For example:

   A40   Streptococcal sepsis
       Code first: postprocedural streptococcal sepsis (T81.4)
                        streptococcal sepsis during labor (O75.3)
                        streptococcal sepsis following abortion or ectopic or molar pregnancy (O03-O07, O08.0)
                        streptococcal sepsis following immunization (T88.0)
                        streptococcal sepsis following infusion, transfusion or therapeutic injection (T80.2)

Hepatitis

The structure of the codes for viral hepatitis has changed. In ICD-9-CM (category 070), fifth digits indicate whether the viral hepatitis is acute or chronic and whether it is associated with hepatitis delta. For example:

070   Viral hepatitis
        The following fifth-digit subclassification is for use with categories 070.2 and 070.3:
        0   Acute or unspecified, without mention of hepatitis delta
        1   Acute or unspecified, with hepatitis delta
        2   Chronic, without mention of hepatitis delta
        3   Chronic, with hepatitis delta

ICD-10-CM includes different category codes to indicate whether the hepatitis is acute or chronic and fourth characters to indicate whether the delta agent is present or absent. For example:

B15   Acute hepatitis A
      B15.0   Hepatitis A with hepatic coma
      B15.9   Hepatitis A without hepatic coma
B16   Acute hepatitis B
      B16.0   Acute hepatitis B with delta-agent with hepatic coma
      B16.1   Acute hepatitis B with delta-agent without hepatic coma
      B16.2   Acute hepatitis B without delta-agent with hepatic coma
      B16.9   Acute hepatitis B without delta-agent and without hepatic coma
B17   Other acute viral hepatitis
      B17.0   Acute delta-(super) infection of hepatitis B carrier
      B17.1   Acute hepatitis C
      B17.2   Acute hepatitis E
      B17.8   Other specified acute viral hepatitis
B18   Chronic viral hepatitis
      B18.0   Chronic viral hepatitis B with delta-agent
      B18.1   Chronic viral hepatitis B without delta-agent
      B18.2   Chronic viral hepatitis C
      B18.8   Other chronic viral hepatitis
      B18.9   Chronic viral hepatitis, unspecified
B19   Unspecified viral hepatitis
      B19.0   Unspecified viral hepatitis with coma
      B19.1   Unspecified viral hepatitis C
             B19.10   Unspecified viral hepatitis C without hepatic coma
             B19.11   Unspecified viral hepatitis C with hepatic coma
      B19.9   Unspecified viral hepatitis without coma

Infectious Mononucleosis

The codes for infectious mononucleosis have been greatly expanded in ICD-10-CM. Fourth characters describe the type of mononucleosis, and fifth characters identify the manifestations. For example:

ICD-9-CM: 075   Infectious mononucleosis
ICD-10-CM: B27   Infectious mononucleosis
                 B27.0   Gammaherpesviral mononucleosis
                     B27.00 Gammaherpesviral mononucleosis without complication
                     B27.01 Gammaherpesviral mononucleosis with polyneuropathy
                     B27.02 Gammaherpesviral mononucleosis with meningitis
                     B27.09 Gammaherpesviral mononucleosis with other complications

The other fourth-character subcategory codes are B27.1, Cytomegaloviral mononucleosis; B27.8, Other infectious mononucleosis; and B27.9, Infectious mononucleosis, unspecified. The fifth characters are the same as in B27.0.

Malaria

ICD-9-CM category 084, Malaria, has been expanded into categories B50 through B54 in ICD-10-CM. The specific categories include:

B50 Plasmodium falciparum malaria
B51 Plasmodium vivax malaria
B52 Plasmodium malariae malaria
B53 Other specified malaria
B54 Unspecified malaria

Fourth characters identify the complications associated with malaria. For example:

B51 Plasmodium vivax malaria
    B51.0 Plasmodium vivax malaria with rupture of spleen
    B51.8 Plasmodium vivax malaria with other complications
    B51.9 Plasmodium vivax malaria without complication

Chagas' Disease

The category for Chagas' disease (B57) has been expanded in ICD-10-CM to identify the associated organ involvement. For example:

B57.0 Acute Chagas' disease with heart involvement
B57.1 Acute Chagas' disease without heart involvement
B57.2 Chagas' disease (chronic) with heart involvement
B57.3 Chagas' disease (chronic) with digestive system involvement
    B57.30 Chagas' disease with digestive system involvement, unspecified
    B57.31 Megaesophagus in Chagas' disease
    B57.32 Megacolon in Chagas' disease
    B57.39 Other digestive system involvement in Chagas' disease
B57.4 Chagas' disease (chronic) with nervous system involvement
    B57.40 Chagas' disease with nervous system involvement, unspecified
    B57.41 Meningitis in Chagas' disease
    B57.42 Meningoencephalitis in Chagas' disease
    B57.49 Other nervous system involvement in Chagas' disease
B57.5 Chagas' disease (chronic) with other organ involvement

Changes in Terminology

The terminology used to describe some infectious diseases has been changed for ICD-10-CM.

Leprosy

The coding professional should note a change in terminology in regard to leprosy. The descriptions of the various types of leprosy have changed between ICD-9-CM category 030, Leprosy, and ICD-10-CM category A30, Leprosy [Hansen's disease]. Physicians should be made aware of these changes and asked to provide specific documentation on the type of leprosy involved.

A30 Leprosy [Hansen's disease]
    A30.0   Indeterminate leprosy
             I leprosy
    A30.1   Tuberculoid leprosy
             TT leprosy
    A30.2   Borderline tuberculoid leprosy
             BT leprosy
    A30.3   Borderline leprosy
             BB leprosy
    A30.4   Borderline lepromatous leprosy
             BL leprosy
    A30.5   Lepromatous leprosy
             LL leprosy
    A30.8   Other forms of leprosy
    A30.9   Leprosy, unspecified

Poliomyelitis

In ICD-10-CM, Acute poliomyelitis, category A80, is described differently than in ICD-9-CM (045). Fifth digits to identify the type of poliovirus (I, II, or III) have been eliminated, and the types of acute paralytic poliomyelitis are identified as vaccine associated (A80.0), imported wild virus (A80.1), or indigenous wild virus (A80.2).

Smallpox

A note under code B03, Smallpox, indicates that the Thirty-third World Health Assembly declared that smallpox had been eradicated, but the code was maintained for surveillance purposes.

Chapter 2

Neoplasms

Chapter 2 in the ICD-10-CM Tabular List classifies neoplastic diseases. It includes categories C00 through D49, which are grouped in the following blocks:

C00–C75	Malignant neoplasms, stated or presumed to be primary, of specified sites, except of lymphoid, hematopoietic and related tissue

	C00–C14	Lip, oral cavity and pharynx
	C15–C26	Digestive organs
	C30–C39	Respiratory and intrathoracic organs
	C40–C41	Bone and articular cartilage
	C43–C44	Skin
	C45–C49	Mesothelial and soft tissue
	C50	Breast
	C51–C58	Female genital organs
	C60–C63	Male genital organs
	C64–C68	Urinary tract
	C69–C72	Eye, brain and other parts of central nervous system
	C73–C75	Thyroid and other endocrine glands

C76–C80	Malignant neoplasms of ill-defined, secondary and unspecified sites
C81–C96	Malignant neoplasms, stated or presumed to be primary, of lymphoid, hematopoietic and related tissue
D00–D09	In situ neoplasms
D10–D36	Benign neoplasms
D37–D48	Neoplasms of uncertain behavior
D49	Neoplasms of unspecified behavior

Title Changes

Chapter 2 of the ICD-10-CM Tabular List includes a number of block and category title changes. A few examples of these changes include the following:

ICD-9-CM:	154	Malignant neoplasm of rectum, rectosigmoid junction and anus
ICD-10-CM:	C19	Malignant neoplasm of rectosigmoid junction

ICD-9-CM:	174	Malignant neoplasm of female breast
	175	Malignant neoplasm of male breast
ICD-10-CM:	C50	Malignant neoplasm of breast

ICD-9-CM:	179	Malignant neoplasm of uterus, part unspecified
	180	Malignant neoplasm of cervix uteri
	181	Malignant neoplasm of placenta
ICD-10-CM:	C51–C58	Malignant neoplasm of female genital organs

Additions, Deletions, and Combinations

When chapter 2 in ICD-10-CM is compared with similar codes in ICD-9-CM, it is evident that many codes have been added, deleted, combined, or moved to another section or chapter. For example, Waldenstrom's macroglobulinemia (273.3) in chapter 3 of ICD-9-CM has been moved to C88, Malignant immunoproliferative diseases, in chapter 2 of ICD-10-CM. This type of change should not present a problem for coding professionals because the Alphabetic Index will direct them to the correct code.

In some instances, codes have been moved from one section to another. For example, in ICD-9-CM, the classification for malignant neoplasms of the retroperitoneum and peritoneum falls within the subchapter entitled Malignant Neoplasm of Digestive Organs and Peritoneum (150–159). In ICD-10-CM, these codes are located in a subchapter entitled Malignant neoplasms of mesothelial and soft tissue (C45–C49).

In ICD-9-CM, the specific codes for cervical, thoracic, and abdominal sites under category 150, Malignant neoplasm of esophagus, have been deleted in ICD-10-CM.

ICD-9-CM:	150	Malignant neoplasm of esophagus
	150.0	Cervical esophagus
	150.1	Thoracic esophagus
	150.2	Abdominal esophagus
	150.3	Upper third of esophagus
	150.4	Middle third of esophagus
	150.5	Lower third of esophagus
	150.8	Other specified part
	150.9	Esophagus, unspecified
ICD-10-CM:	C15	Malignant neoplasm of esophagus
	C15.3	Malignant neoplasm of upper third of esophagus
	C15.4	Malignant neoplasm of middle third of esophagus
	C15.5	Malignant neoplasm of lower third of esophagus
	C15.8	Malignant neoplasm of overlapping sites of esophagus
	C15.9	Malignant neoplasm of esophagus, unspecified

In ICD-10-CM, category C38, Malignant neoplasm of heart, mediastinum and pleura, contains a subcategory C38.4, Malignant neoplasm of pleura, which differs from the ICD-9-CM category 163, Malignant neoplasm of pleura. ICD-9-CM specifically lists codes for parietal pleura, visceral pleura, other specified sites of pleura, and pleura, unspecified, which have been deleted from ICD-10-CM.

ICD-9-CM: 163   Malignant neoplasm of pleura
- 163.0   Parietal pleura
- 163.1   Visceral pleura
- 163.8   Other specified sites of pleura
- 163.9   Pleura, unspecified

ICD-10-CM: C38   Malignant neoplasm of heart, mediastinum and pleura
- C38.0   Malignant neoplasm of heart
- C38.1   Malignant neoplasm of anterior mediastinum
- C38.2   Malignant neoplasm of posterior mediastinum
- C38.3   Malignant neoplasm of mediastinum, part unspecified
- C38.4   Malignant neoplasm of pleura
- C38.8   Malignant neoplasm of overlapping sites of heart, mediastinum and pleura

In ICD-10-CM, category D03, Melanoma in situ, has been added as a new category. In ICD-9-CM, melanoma in situ is included in category 172, Malignant melanoma of skin.

Expansions and Consolidations

A number of codes for neoplastic diseases have been expanded in ICD-10-CM. For example, the code for carcinoma in situ of skin (232) in ICD-9-CM has been expanded in ICD-10-CM to fifth characters to indicate specific sites and laterality.

ICD-9-CM: 232   Carcinoma in situ of skin
- 232.0   Eyelid, including canthus
- 232.1   Ear and external auditory canal
- 232.3   Skin of other and unspecified parts of face
- 232.4   Scalp and skin of neck
- 232.5   Skin of trunk, except scrotum
- 232.6   Skin of upper limb, including shoulder
- 232.7   Skin of lower limb, including hip
- 232.8   Other specified sites of skin
- 232.9   Skin, site unspecified

ICD-10-CM: D04   Carcinoma in situ of skin
- D04.0   Carcinoma in situ of skin of lip
- D04.1   Carcinoma in situ of skin of eyelid, including canthus
  - D04.10   Carcinoma in situ of skin of eyelid, including canthus, unspecified side
  - D04.11   Carcinoma in situ of skin of right eyelid, including canthus
  - D04.12   Carcinoma in situ of skin of left eyelid, including canthus
- D04.2   Carcinoma in situ of skin of ear and external auricular canal
  - D04.20   Carcinoma in situ of skin of ear and external auricular canal, unspecified side
  - D04.21   Carcinoma in situ of skin of right ear and external auricular canal
  - D04.22   Carcinoma in situ of skin of left ear and external auricular canal
- D04.3   Carcinoma in situ of skin of other and unspecified parts of face
  - D04.30   Carcinoma in situ of skin of unspecified part of face
  - D04.39   Carcinoma in situ of skin of other parts of face

D04.4	Carcinoma in situ of skin of scalp and neck
D04.5	Carcinoma in situ of skin of trunk
D04.6	Carcinoma in situ of skin of upper limb, including shoulder

	D04.60	Carcinoma in situ of skin of upper limb, including shoulder, unspecified side
	D04.61	Carcinoma in situ of skin of right upper limb, including shoulder
	D04.62	Carcinoma in situ of skin of left upper limb, including shoulder

| D04.7 | Carcinoma in situ of skin of lower limb, including hip |

	D04.70	Carcinoma in situ of skin of lower limb, including hip, unspecified side
	D04.71	Carcinoma in situ of skin of right lower limb, including hip
	D04.72	Carcinoma in situ of skin of left lower limb, including hip

| D04.8 | Carcinoma in situ of skin of other sites |
| D04.9 | Carcinoma in situ of skin, unspecified |

ICD-9-CM category 189, Malignant neoplasm of kidney and other and unspecified urinary organs, has been split into four category codes in ICD-10-CM: C64, Malignant neoplasm of kidney, except renal pelvis; C65, Malignant neoplasm of renal pelvis; C66, Malignant neoplasm of ureter; C67, Malignant neoplasm of bladder; and C68, Malignant neoplasm of other and unspecified urinary organs.

Some codes have been restructured with consolidation of some categories. For example, ICD-9-CM category codes 174, Malignant neoplasm of female breast, and 175, Malignant neoplasm of male breast, have been consolidated into C50, Malignant neoplasm of breast.

In numerous instances, codes included as subcategory codes in ICD-9-CM have been given a specific category code in ICD-10-CM and expanded to the fourth- or fifth-character level. For example:

| ICD-9-CM: | 202.0 | Nodular lymphoma |
| ICD-10-CM: | C82 | Follicular [nodular] non-Hodgkin's lymphoma |

| | C82.0 | Small cleaved cell, follicular non-Hodgkin's lymphoma |

	C82.00	Small cleaved cell, follicular non-Hodgkin's lymphoma, unspecified site
	C82.01	Small cleaved cell, follicular non-Hodgkin's lymphoma, lymph nodes of head, face, and neck
	C82.02	Small cleaved cell, follicular non-Hodgkin's lymphoma, intrathoracic lymph nodes
	C82.03	Small cleaved cell, follicular non-Hodgkin's lymphoma, intra-abdominal lymph nodes
	C82.04	Small cleaved cell, follicular non-Hodgkin's lymphoma, lymph nodes of axilla and upper limb
	C82.05	Small cleaved cell, follicular non-Hodgkin's lymphoma, lymph nodes of inguinal region and lower limb
	C82.06	Small cleaved cell, follicular non-Hodgkin's lymphoma, intrapelvic lymph nodes
	C82.07	Small cleaved cell, follicular non-Hodgkin's lymphoma, spleen
	C82.08	Small cleaved cell, follicular non-Hodgkin's lymphoma, lymph nodes of multiple sites
	C82.09	Small cleaved cell, follicular non-Hodgkin's lymphoma, extranodal and solid organ sites

ICD-9-CM: 202.1   Mycosis fungoides
ICD-10-CM: C84   Peripheral and cutaneous T-cell lymphomas
                 C84.0 Mycosis fungoides

C84.00	Mycosis fungoides, unspecified site
C84.01	Mycosis fungoides, lymph nodes of head, face and neck
C84.02	Mycosis fungoides, intrathoracic lymph nodes
C84.03	Mycosis fungoides, intra-abdominal lymph nodes
C84.04	Mycosis fungoides, lymph nodes of axilla and upper limb
C84.05	Mycosis fungoides, lymph nodes of inguinal region and lower limb
C84.06	Mycosis fungoides, intrapelvic lymph nodes
C84.07	Mycosis fungoides, spleen
C84.08	Mycosis fungoides, lymph nodes of multiple sites
C84.09	Mycosis fungoides, extranodal and solid organ sites

Neoplasms of uncertain behavior in ICD-10-CM have been expanded to include fifth and, in some cases, even sixth characters to further specify sites or organs. Changes in these categories should be conveyed to physicians to make them aware of the documentation needed for accurate coding.

Carcinoma in Situ of Breast

In ICD-9-CM, carcinoma in situ of breast (233.0) is described differently in ICD-10-CM (D05). A separate category code is assigned to this condition, and fourth and fifth characters are used to further describe lobular, intraductal, other, and unspecified carcinoma in situ of the breast. At the fifth-character level, female versus male breast is differentiated as well as laterality of each.

Expansion of Category Codes

ICD-10-CM includes category codes that specify the use of additional codes to identify the following: alcohol abuse and dependence (F10.–), alcohol dependence in remission (F10.21), history of tobacco use (Z87.82), tobacco dependence (F17.–), and tobacco use (Z72.0). Examples of these category codes include C00 through C06. In addition, categories C07 through C10 require the coding professional to further identify exposure to environmental tobacco smoke (Z58.83), exposure to tobacco smoke in the perinatal period (P96.6), and occupational exposure to environmental tobacco smoke (Z57.31). Category C22 further requires the coding professional to identify hepatitis B (B16.–, B18.0–B18.1) and hepatitis C (B17.1, B18.2).

A number of ICD-10-CM categories include notes to indicate that morphology codes must be included with behavior code/3. Examples are categories C45, Mesothelioma; C46, Kaposi's sarcoma; and categories C81 through C96.

Hodgkin's Disease

The codes for Hodgkin's disease, block C81, have been expanded in ICD-10-CM with fourth characters that indicate the various types and fifth characters that specify lymph node involvement. An additional subdivision (extranodal and solid organ sites) has been added in ICD-10-CM. Categories C82, Follicular [nodular] non-Hodgkin's lymphoma, and C83, Diffuse non-Hodgkin's lymphoma, have been expanded in a similar manner.

Chapter 3

Diseases of the Blood and Blood-Forming Organs and Disorders of the Immune System

Chapter 3 of the ICD-10-CM Tabular List classifies diseases of the blood and blood-forming organs and certain disorders involving the immune mechanism. It includes categories D50 through D89, which are arranged in the following blocks:

D50–D53   Nutritional anemias
D55–D59   Hemolytic anemias
D60–D64   Aplastic and other anemias
D65–D69   Coagulation defects, purpura and other hemorrhagic conditions
D70–D78   Other diseases of blood and blood-forming organs
D80–D89   Certain disorders involving the immune mechanism

Chapter 3 of ICD-10-CM includes codes primarily from ICD-9-CM chapter 4, Diseases of the Blood and Blood-Forming Organs, but also includes many codes from chapter 3, Endocrine, Nutritional and Metabolic Diseases and Immunity Disorders. ICD-10-CM chapter 3 also includes some codes from ICD-9-CM chapter 1, Infectious and Parasitic Diseases. One such example is sarcoidosis (D86). For the most part, the codes in block D80 through D89 were previously included in chapter 3 of ICD-9-CM.

Title Changes

There have been a number of block and category title changes in chapter 3 of ICD-10-CM. A few examples of these changes include:

ICD-9-CM: 281.0   Pernicious anemia
ICD-10-CM: D51.0   Vitamin B_{12} deficiency anemia due to intrinsic factor deficiency

ICD-9-CM: 282.2   Anemias due to disorders of glutathione metabolism
ICD-10-CM: D55   Anemia due to enzyme disorders

Additions, Deletions, and Combinations

When chapter 3 of ICD-10-CM is compared with chapter 4 in ICD-9-CM, it is evident that some codes have been added, deleted, combined, or moved from one section or chapter to another. For example, in ICD-9-CM, sickle-cell thalassemia is classified to code 282.4, Thalassemias. In ICD-10-CM, sickle-cell thalassemia is classified to D57, Sickle-cell disorders. The correct code assignment would be D57.40, Sickle-cell thalassemia.

Expansions

A number of codes for diseases of the blood and blood-forming organs and disorders of the immune system have been expanded in ICD-10-CM.

Expansions to Increase Specificity

There is increased specificity in many of the blocks/codes in ICD-10-CM. This increased specificity means that coding professionals will have to review the record carefully to find the needed information. Further, physicians will have to document more information about the types of anemias. A few examples that demonstrate this increased specificity include:

ICD-9-CM:	282.2	Anemias due to disorders of glutathione metabolism
ICD-10-CM:	D55	Anemia due to enzyme disorders
	D55.0	Anemia due to glucose-6-phosphate dehydrogenase [G6PD] deficiency
	D55.1	Anemia due to other disorders of glutathione metabolism
	D55.2	Anemia due to disorders of glycolytic enzymes
	D55.3	Anemia due to disorders of nucleotide metabolism
	D55.8	Other anemias due to enzyme disorders
	D55.9	Anemia due to enzyme disorder, unspecified

ICD-9-CM:	282.4	Thalassemias
ICD-10-CM:	D56	Thalassemia

Excludes 1: sickle-cell thalassemia (D57.4)

	D56.0	Alpha thalassemia
	D56.1	Beta thalassemia
	D56.2	Delta-beta thalassemia
	D56.3	Thalassemia minor
	D56.4	Hereditary persistence of fetal hemoglobin [HPFH]
	D56.8	Other thalassemias
	D56.9	Thalassemia, unspecified

ICD-9-CM:	284.8	Other specified aplastic anemias
ICD-10-CM:	D61	Other aplastic anemias
	D61.0	Constitutional aplastic anemia
	D61.1	Drug-induced aplastic anemia
	D61.2	Aplastic anemia due to other external agents
	D61.3	Idiopathic aplastic anemia
	D61.4	Congenital red cell aplasia
	D61.8	Other specified aplastic anemias
	D61.9	Aplastic anemia, unspecified

ICD-9-CM:	288.0	Agranulocytosis
ICD-10-CM:	D70	Neutropenia
	D70.0	Congenital agranulocytosis
	D70.1	Agranulocytosis secondary to cancer chemotherapy
	D70.2	Other drug-induced agranulocytosis
	D70.3	Other agranulocytosis
	D70.4	Cyclic neutropenia
	D70.8	Other neutropenia
	D70.9	Neutropenia, unspecified

The codes for conditions of the spleen have added specificity in ICD-10-CM. In addition to the added specificity, a new code is assigned to report intraoperative and postprocedural complications of procedures on the spleen.

D78   Intraoperative and postprocedural complications of procedures on the spleen
    D78.0   Intraoperative and postprocedural hemorrhage or hematoma complicating procedures on the spleen
            Excludes 1: intraoperative hemorrhage or hematoma due to accidental puncture or laceration during a procedure on the spleen (D78.1–)
    D78.1   Accidental puncture or laceration during a procedure on the spleen
    D78.8   Other intraoperative and postprocedural complications of procedures on the spleen

Each of these four-character codes has fifth characters that provide additional specificity. An example from each of the fourth characters includes:

D78.01   Intraoperative hemorrhage of the spleen during a procedure on the spleen
D78.12   Accidental puncture or laceration of other organ or structure during a procedure on the spleen
D78.81   Other intraoperative complications of procedures on the spleen

Disorders Involving the Immune Mechanism

The last block in this chapter (D80–D89) groups disorders involving the immune mechanism. The various rubrics included in this block are:

D80   Immunodeficiency with predominantly antibody defects
D81   Combined immunodeficiencies
D82   Immunodeficiency associated with other major defects
D83   Common variable immunodeficiency
D84   Other immunodeficiencies
D86   Sarcoidosis
D89   Other disorders involving the immune mechanism, not elsewhere classified

Many of these codes have increased specificity at the fourth-, fifth-, or sixth-character level. For example:

ICD-9-CM: 279.06   Common variable immunodeficiency
ICD-10-CM: D83   Common variable immunodeficiency
        D83.0   Common variable immunodeficiency with predominant abnormalities of B-cell numbers and function
        D83.1   Common variable immunodeficiency with predominant immunoregulatory T-cell disorders
        D83.2   Common variable immunodeficiency with autoantibodies to B- or T-cells
        D83.8   Other common variable immunodeficiencies
        D83.9   Common variable immunodeficiency, unspecified

Chapter 4

Endocrine, Nutritional, and Metabolic Diseases

Chapter 4 of the ICD-10-CM Tabular List classifies certain endocrine, nutritional, and metabolic diseases. It includes categories E00 through E90, which are arranged in the following blocks:

E00–E07   Disorders of thyroid gland
E08–E14   Diabetes mellitus
E15–E16   Other disorders of glucose regulation and pancreatic internal secretion
E20–E36   Disorders of other endocrine glands
E40–E46   Malnutrition
E50–E64   Other nutritional deficiencies
E65–E68   Obesity and other hyperalimentation
E70–E89   Metabolic disorders

Title Changes

A number of block and category title changes have been made in chapter 4 of ICD-10-CM. A few examples of these changes include the following:

ICD-9-CM: Nutritional Deficiencies (260–269)
ICD-10-CM: Malnutrition (E40–E46)

ICD-9-CM: 259   Other endocrine disorders
ICD-10-CM: E30   Disorders of puberty, not elsewhere classified

ICD-9-CM: 252   Disorders of parathyroid gland
ICD-10-CM: E20   Hypoparathyroidism

Additions, Deletions, and Combinations

When chapter 4 of ICD-10-CM is compared with chapter 3 of ICD-9-CM, it is evident that many codes have been added, deleted, combined, or moved to another section or chapter. Examples of codes that have been moved to chapter 4 of ICD-10-CM include 330.1, Cerebral lipidoses, from chapter 6, Diseases of the Nervous System and Sense Organs, in ICD-9-CM; and Smith-Lemli-Opitz syndrome (E78.72), from chapter 14, Congenital Anomalies, in ICD-9-CM.

A new category in ICD-10-CM called Drug or chemical induced diabetes mellitus (E09) includes the following subcategories:

E09   Drug or chemical induced diabetes mellitus
       Code first (T36–T65) to identify drug or chemical
       Use additional code to identify any insulin use (Z79.7)
       E09.0   Drug or chemical induced diabetes mellitus with hyperosmolarity
       E09.1   Drug or chemical induced diabetes mellitus with ketoacidosis
       E09.2   Drug or chemical induced diabetes mellitus with renal complications
       E09.3   Drug or chemical induced diabetes mellitus with ophthalmic complications
       E09.4   Drug or chemical induced diabetes mellitus with neurological complications
       E09.5   Drug or chemical induced diabetes mellitus with circulatory complications
       E09.6   Drug or chemical induced diabetes mellitus with other specified complications
       E09.8   Drug or chemical induced diabetes mellitus with unspecified complications
       E09.9   Drug or chemical induced diabetes mellitus without complications

Fifth and sixth characters under this category indicate specific manifestations of the listed complication(s).

Another new section in chapter 4 of ICD-10-CM is E36, Intraoperative and postprocedural complications of endocrine procedures. This section includes the following codes:

E36.0   Intraoperative and postprocedural hemorrhage or hematoma complicating an endocrine
         procedure
         E36.01   Intraoperative hemorrhage of an endocrine organ during an endocrine
                   procedure
         E36.02   Intraoperative hemorrhage of other organ during an endocrine procedure
         E36.03   Intraoperative hematoma of an endocrine organ during an endocrine procedure
         E36.04   Intraoperative hematoma of other organ during an endocrine procedure
         E36.05   Postprocedural hemorrhage of an endocrine organ following an endocrine
                   procedure
         E36.06   Postprocedural hemorrhage of other organ following an endocrine procedure
         E36.07   Postprocedural hematoma of an endocrine organ following an endocrine
                   procedure
         E36.08   Postprocedural hematoma of other organ following an endocrine procedure
E36.1   Accidental puncture or laceration of an endocrine organ during an endocrine procedure
         E36.11   Accidental puncture or laceration of an endocrine organ during an endocrine
                   procedure
         E36.12   Accidental puncture or laceration of other organs during an endocrine procedure
E36.8   Other intraoperative and postprocedural complications of endocrine procedures
         E36.81   Other intraoperative complications of endocrine procedures
         E36.89   Other postprocedural complications of endocrine procedures

ICD-9-CM does not list a separate code for hypovolemia or dehydration. These two conditions along with depletion of volume of plasma or extracellular fluid are grouped into subcategory code 276.5, Volume depletion. In ICD-10-CM, these conditions are classified independently. For example:

ICD-9-CM: 276.5   Volume depletion
ICD-10-CM: E86   Volume depletion
                     E86.0   Dehydration
                     E86.1   Hypovolemia
                     E86.9   Volume depletion, unspecified

Expansions

The ICD-9-CM code for hypoparathyroidism (252.1) has been expanded in ICD-10-CM, as follows:

E20   Hypoparathyroidism
    E20.0   Idiopathic hypoparathyroidism
    E20.1   Pseudohypoparathyroidism
    E20.8   Other hypoparathyroidism
    E20.9   Hypoparathyroidism, unspecified

The code for beriberi (E51.1) has been expanded to fifth characters to indicate specific types of beriberi. For example:

ICD-9-CM: 265.1   Beriberi
ICD-10-CM: E51.1   Beriberi
                E51.11   Dry beriberi
                E51.12   Wet beriberi

Diabetes Mellitus

ICD-9-CM category 250, Diabetes mellitus, has been split into six category codes in ICD-10-CM:

E08   Diabetes mellitus due to underlying condition
E09   Drug or chemical induced diabetes mellitus
E10   Type 1 diabetes mellitus
E11   Type 2 diabetes mellitus
E13   Other specified diabetes mellitus
E14   Unspecified diabetes mellitus

All of these categories, with the exception of category E10, have a note that directs users to use an additional code to identify any insulin use (Z79.7). Fourth characters under these categories refer to underlying conditions with specified complications, fifth characters define the specific manifestation (ketoacidosis, nephropathy, neuropathy, peripheral angiopathy), and sixth characters define the manifestation even further. For example:

E11   Type 2 diabetes mellitus
    E11.0   Type 2 diabetes mellitus with hyperosmolarity
        E11.00   Type 2 diabetes mellitus with hyperosmolarity without nonketotic hyperglycemic-hyperosmolar coma (NKHHC)
        E11.01   Type 2 diabetes mellitus with hyperosmolarity with coma
    E11.6   Type 2 diabetes mellitus with other specified complications
        E11.61   Type 2 diabetes mellitus with diabetic arthropathy
            E11.610   Type 2 diabetes mellitus with diabetic neuropathic arthropathy
            E11.618   Type 2 diabetes mellitus with other diabetic arthropathy

In numerous instances, codes included as subcategory codes in ICD-9-CM have been given a specific category code in ICD-10-CM and expanded at the fourth- or fifth-character level. For example:

ICD-9-CM:	278.00	Obesity
	278.01	Morbid obesity
ICD-10-CM:	E66	Obesity

        E66.0   Obesity due to excess calories
                E66.01   Morbid obesity due to excess calories
                E66.09   Other obesity due to excess calories
        E66.1   Drug-induced obesity
        E66.2   Morbid (severe) obesity with alveolar hypoventilation
        E66.8   Other obesity
        E66.9   Obesity, unspecified

Changes in these categories should be conveyed to physicians to make them aware of the documentation needed for accurate coding.

Expansions to Reflect Manifestations

Some of the codes in ICD-10-CM chapter 4 have been expanded to reflect manifestations of the disease by using fourth or fifth characters rather than by using an additional code to identify the manifestation. For example:

| ICD-9-CM: | 250.4 | Diabetes with renal manifestations |

Use additional code to identify manifestation as:
    diabetic:
        nephropathy, not otherwise specified (583.81)
        nephrosis (581.81)
    intercapillary glomerulosclerosis (581.81)
    Kimmelstiel-Wilson syndrome (581.81)

| ICD-10-CM: | E08.2 | Diabetes mellitus due to underlying condition with renal complications |

        E08.21   Diabetes mellitus due to underlying condition with diabetic nephropathy
        E08.22   Diabetes mellitus due to underlying condition with Ebstein's disease
        E08.23   Diabetes mellitus due to underlying condition with diabetic renal failure
        E08.29   Diabetes mellitus due to underlying condition with other diabetic renal complication

Expansions to Include Notes

In some instances in ICD-10-CM, notes have been added to a category or subcategory code to indicate that the code can be used as an additional code to identify functional activity. For example:

| ICD-9-CM: | 259.2 | Carcinoid syndrome |
| ICD-10-CM: | E34.0 | Carcinoid syndrome |

        Note: May be used as an additional code to identify functional activity associated with a carcinoid tumor.

ICD-9-CM subcategory 269.3, Mineral deficiency, not elsewhere classified, has been expanded in ICD-10-CM into categories E58, Dietary calcium deficiency; E59, Dietary selenium deficiency; and E60, Dietary zinc deficiency.

Expansion to Fifth and Sixth Characters

Another example of expansion in ICD-10-CM includes a subcategory code that has been expanded to include not only fifth, but also sixth characters:

ICD-9-CM:	270.2	Other disturbances of aromatic amino-acid metabolism
ICD-10-CM:	E70.0	Classical phenylketonuria
	E70.1	Other hyperphenylalaninemias
	E70.2	Disorders of tyrosine metabolism

E70.20	Disorder of tyrosine metabolism, unspecified
E70.21	Tyrosinemia
E70.29	Other disorders of tyrosine metabolism

E70.3   Albinism

E70.30	Albinism, unspecified
E70.31	Ocular albinism

E70.310	X-linked ocular albinism
E70.311	Autosomal recessive ocular albinism
E70.318	Other ocular albinism
E70.319	Ocular albinism, unspecified

E70.32   Oculocutaneous albinism

E70.320	Tyrosinase negative oculocutaneous albinism
E70.321	Tyrosinase positive oculocutaneous albinism
E70.328	Other oculocutaneous albinism
E70.329	Oculocutaneous albinism, unspecified

E70.33   Albinism with hematologic abnormality

E70.330	Chediak-Higashi syndrome
E70.331	Hemansky-Pudlak syndrome
E70.338	Other albinism with hematologic abnormality
E70.339	Albinism with hematologic abnormality, unspecified

E70.39	Other specified albinism

E70.4   Disorders of histidine metabolism

E70.40	Disorders of histidine metabolism, unspecified
E70.41	Histidinemia
E70.49	Other disorders of histidine metabolism

E70.5	Disorders of tryptophan metabolism
E70.8	Other disorders of aromatic amino-acid metabolism
E70.9	Disorder of aromatic amino-acid metabolism, unspecified

Chapter 5

Mental and Behavioral Disorders

Chapter 5 in the ICD-10-CM Tabular List classifies mental and behavioral disorders. It includes categories F01 through F99, which are arranged in the following blocks:

F01–F09   Mental disorders due to known physiological conditions

F10–F19   Mental and behavioral disorders due to psychoactive substance use

F20–F29   Schizophrenia, schizotypal and delusional, and other non-mood psychotic disorders

F30–F39   Mood [affective] disorders

F40–F48   Anxiety, dissociative, stress-related, somatoform and other nonpsychotic mental disorders

F50–F59   Behavioral syndromes associated with physiological disturbances and physical factors

F60–F69   Disorders of adult personality and behavior

F70–F79   Mental retardation

F80–F89   Pervasive and specific developmental disorders

F90–F98   Behavioral and emotional disorders with onset usually occurring in childhood and adolescence

F99   Unspecified mental disorder

The arrangement of the codes within the various blocks is significantly different in ICD-10-CM compared to ICD-9-CM, although the actual codes remain similar.

Title Changes

A number of block and category title changes have been made in chapter 5 of ICD-10-CM. A few examples of these changes include the following:

ICD-9-CM:	296.0	Manic disorder, single episode
ICD-10-CM:	F30	Manic episode
ICD-9-CM:	308	Acute reaction to stress
ICD-10-CM:	F43	Reaction to severe stress, and adjustment disorders

There are no significant changes in the titles or uses of codes in blocks F80 through F89, Pervasive and specific developmental disorders, and F90 through F98, Behavioral and emotional disorders with onset usually occurring in childhood and adolescence. Likewise, the codes in blocks F60 through F69, Disorders of adult personality and behavior, are very similar to those in ICD-9-CM.

Additions, Deletions, and Combinations

When chapter 5 of ICD-10-CM is compared with chapter 5 in ICD-9-CM, it is evident that some codes have been added, deleted, combined, or moved to another section or chapter. For example, in ICD-10-CM, category F55, Abuse of non-psychoactive substances, includes abuse of antacids, herbal or folk remedies, laxatives, steroids or hormones, and vitamins. In ICD-9-CM, this abuse is grouped with nondependent abuse of drugs.

Expansions

A number of codes for mental and behavioral disorders have been expanded in ICD-10-CM.

Mental and Behavioral Disorders Due to Psychoactive Substance Use

Codes in F10 through F19, Mental and behavioral disorders due to psychoactive substance use, classify alcohol-related and substance-related abuse and dependence that are classified to categories 303 through 305 in ICD-9-CM. These codes have been greatly expanded in ICD-10-CM.

A *use additional code* note under category F10, Alcohol-related disorders, reminds the coding professional that an additional code to identify blood alcohol level (Y90.–) may be used, if applicable. Fourth characters in F10 differentiate between alcohol abuse (F10.1), alcohol dependence (F10.2), and unspecified alcohol use (F10.9). Fifth and sixth characters provide greater specificity. For example:

F10.1 Alcohol abuse
Excludes 1: alcohol dependence (F10.2–)
alcohol use, unspecified (F10.9–)
F10.10 Alcohol abuse, uncomplicated
F10.12 Alcohol abuse with intoxication
F10.120 Alcohol abuse with intoxication, uncomplicated
F10.121 Alcohol abuse with intoxication delirium
F10.129 Alcohol abuse with intoxication, unspecified
F10.14 Alcohol abuse with alcohol-induced mood disorder
F10.15 Alcohol abuse with alcohol-induced psychotic disorder
F10.150 Alcohol abuse with alcohol-induced psychotic disorder with delusions
F10.151 Alcohol abuse with alcohol-induced psychotic disorder with hallucinations
F10.159 Alcohol abuse with alcohol-induced psychotic disorder, unspecified
F10.18 Alcohol abuse with other alcohol-induced disorders
F10.180 Alcohol abuse with alcohol-induced anxiety disorder
F10.181 Alcohol abuse with alcohol-induced sexual dysfunction
F10.182 Alcohol abuse with alcohol-induced sleep disorder
F10.188 Alcohol abuse with other alcohol-induced disorder
F10.19 Alcohol abuse with unspecified alcohol-induced disorder

Codes F11 through F16 identify substance-related disorders such as opioid-related disorders (F11); cannabis-related disorders (F12); sedative, hypnotic, or anxiolytic-related disorders (F13); cocaine-related disorders (F14); other stimulant-related disorders (F15); and hallucinogen-related disorders (F16). Within each of these categories, fourth characters differentiate among abuse, dependence, and unspecified use. Fifth and sixth characters provide greater specificity to generally describe whether the patient is suffering from delusions, hallucinations, perceptual disturbances, sexual dysfunction, sleep disturbances, or other complications. In each category for substance dependence is a code that identifies that the problem is in remission. Some examples of codes from this block include:

F14.2   Cocaine dependence
     Excludes 1:   cocaine abuse (F14.1–)
                    cocaine use, unspecified (F14.9–)
     Excludes 2:   cocaine poisoning (T40.5–)
     F14.20   Cocaine dependence, uncomplicated
     F14.21   Cocaine dependence, in remission
     F14.22   Cocaine dependence with intoxication
            F14.220   Cocaine dependence with intoxication, uncomplicated
            F14.221   Cocaine dependence with intoxication delirium
            F14.222   Cocaine dependence with intoxication with perceptual disturbance
            F14.229   Cocaine dependence with intoxication, unspecified
     F14.23   Cocaine dependence with withdrawal
     F14.24   Cocaine dependence with cocaine-induced mood disorder
     F14.25   Cocaine dependence with cocaine-induced psychotic disorder
            F14.250   Cocaine dependence with cocaine-induced psychotic disorder with delusions
            F14.251   Cocaine dependence with cocaine-induced psychotic disorder with hallucinations
            F14.259   Cocaine dependence with cocaine-induced psychotic disorder, unspecified
     F14.28   Cocaine dependence with other cocaine-induced disorder
            F14.280   Cocaine dependence with cocaine-induced anxiety disorder
            F14.281   Cocaine dependence with cocaine-induced sexual dysfunction
            F14.282   Cocaine dependence with cocaine-induced sleep disorder
            F14.288   Cocaine dependence with other cocaine-induced disorder
     F14.29   Cocaine dependence with unspecified cocaine-induced disorder

Code F17, Nicotine dependence, is subdivided to identify the nicotine product such as cigarettes, chewing tobacco, or other tobacco product. Sixth characters indicate whether the dependence is uncomplicated, in remission, in withdrawal, with other nicotine-induced disorders, or unspecified. Tobacco use not otherwise specified is assigned to category Z72.0, and a history of tobacco dependence is assigned to category Z87.82.

Category F18 is used to report abuse or dependence of inhalant-related disorders with fourth, fifth, and sixth characters similar to the other categories in F10 through F19, Mental and behavioral disorders due to psychoactive substance abuse.

Mood (Affective) Disorders

Fifth characters describing the severity of bipolar disease used in ICD-9-CM are incorporated into category codes F30 through F39, Mood [affective] disorders, in ICD-10-CM at the fourth- and fifth-character levels. For example:

F30   Manic episode
    Includes: bipolar disorder, single manic episode
                   mixed affective episode
    Excludes 1: bipolar disorder (F31.–)
                   major depressive disorder, single episode (F32.–)
                   major depressive disorder, recurrent (F33.–)

    F30.1 Manic episode without psychotic symptoms
        F30.10   Manic episode without psychotic symptoms, unspecified
        F30.11   Manic episode without psychotic symptoms, mild
        F30.12   Manic episode without psychotic symptoms, moderate
        F30.13   Manic episode, severe, without psychotic symptoms
    F30.2 Manic episode, severe with psychotic symptoms
    F30.3 Manic episode in partial remission
    F30.4 Manic episode in full remission
    F30.8 Other manic episodes
    F30.9 Manic episode, unspecified

Other category codes in this section include:

F31   Bipolar disorder

F32   Major depressive disorder, single episode

F33   Major depressive disorder, recurrent

F34   Persistent mood [affective] disorders

F39   Unspecified mood [affective] disorders

Anxiety, Dissociative, Stress-Related, Somatoform, and Other Nonpsychotic Mental Disorders

The codes in F40 through F48, Anxiety, dissociative, stress-related, somatoform and other nonpsychotic mental disorders, have been greatly expanded in ICD-10-CM through the use of fourth, fifth, and sixth characters. This block includes the following categories:

F40   Phobic anxiety disorders

F41   Other anxiety disorders

F42   Obsessive-compulsive disorder

F43   Reaction to severe stress, and adjustment disorders

F44   Dissociative and conversion disorders

F45   Somatoform disorders

F48   Other nonpsychotic mental disorders

An example of one of the codes from this block is:

F40   Phobic anxiety disorders
    F40.0 Agoraphobia
        F40.00   Agoraphobia, unspecified
        F40.01   Agoraphobia with panic disorder
        F40.02   Agoraphobia without panic disorder
    F40.1 Social phobias
        F40.10   Social phobia, unspecified
        F40.11   Social phobia, generalized

F40.2　Specific (isolated) phobias
　　　　F40.21　Animal type phobia
　　　　　　　　F40.210　Arachnophobia
　　　　　　　　F40.218　Other animal type phobia
　　　　F40.22　Natural environment type phobia
　　　　　　　　F40.220　Fear of thunderstorms
　　　　　　　　F40.228　Other natural environment type phobia
　　　　F40.23　Blood, injection, injury type phobia
　　　　　　　　F40.230　Fear of blood
　　　　　　　　F40.231　Fear of injections and transfusions
　　　　　　　　F40.232　Fear of other medical care
　　　　　　　　F40.233　Fear of injury
　　　　F40.24　Situational type phobia
　　　　　　　　F40.240　Claustrophobia
　　　　　　　　F40.241　Acrophobia
　　　　　　　　F40.242　Fear of bridges
　　　　　　　　F40.243　Fear of flying
　　　　　　　　F40.248　Other situational type phobia
　　　　F40.29　Other specified phobia
　　　　　　　　F40.290　Androphobia
　　　　　　　　F40.291　Gynephobia
　　　　　　　　F40.298　Other specified phobia
F40.8　Other phobic anxiety disorders
F40.9　Phobic anxiety disorder, unspecified

Changes in Terminology

Some changes in terminology are included in categories F20 through F29, Schizophrenia, schizotypal, delusional, and other non-mood psychotic disorders. For example, ICD-10-CM category F21, Schizotypal disorder, has an inclusion term for latent schizophrenia, which was listed in ICD-9-CM as code 295.5, Latent schizophrenia. Category 297, Paranoid states (delusional disorders), in ICD-9-CM became F22, Delusional disorders, in ICD-10-CM.

The major change for the types of conditions covered in categories F50 through F59, Behavioral syndromes associated with physiological disturbances and physical factors, is found in F51, Sleep disorders not due to a substance or known physiological condition. ICD-10-CM uses different terminology in describing sleep disorders than is found in ICD-9-CM. For example:

F51.2　Circadian rhythm sleep disorder not due to a substance or known physiological condition
　　　　F51.20　Circadian rhythm sleep disorder not due to a substance or known physiological condition, unspecified type
　　　　F51.21　Circadian rhythm sleep disorder not due to a substance or known physiological condition, jet-lag type
　　　　F51.22　Circadian rhythm sleep disorder not due to a substance or known physiological condition, shift-work type
　　　　F51.23　Circadian rhythm sleep disorder not due to a substance or known physiological condition, delayed sleep phase type
　　　　F51.29　Other sleep disorder of circadian rhythm not due to a substance or known physiological condition

Changes in Directions

A significant change in F70 through F79, Mental retardation, involves the direction to the coding professional to code first any associated physical or developmental disorder. In ICD-9-CM, the coding professional is directed to use additional code(s) to identify any associated psychiatric or physical condition(s).

Categories F01 through F09, Mental disorders due to known physiological conditions, comprise a range of mental disorders grouped together on the basis of their having in common a demonstrable etiology in cerebral disease, brain injury, or other insult leading to cerebral dysfunction. The dysfunction may be primary, as in diseases, injuries, and insults that affect the brain directly and selectively; or secondary, as in systemic diseases and disorders that attack the brain only as one of the multiple organs or systems of the body that are involved. The instructions in the Tabular List indicate that the coding professional should code first the underlying physiological condition.

Some of the codes found in this block include:

F01   Vascular dementia
F02   Dementia in other diseases classified elsewhere
F03   Unspecified dementia
F04   Amnestic disorder due to known physiological condition
F05   Delirium due to known physiological condition
F06   Other mental disorders due to known physiological condition
F07   Personality and behavioral disorders due to known physiological condition
F09   Unspecified mental disorder due to known physiological condition

These codes are further divided into fourth-, fifth-, and sixth-character levels. For example:

F06   Other mental disorders due to known physiological condition
       Includes: mental disorders due to endocrine disorder
                     mental disorders due to exogenous hormone
                     mental disorders due to exogenous toxic substance
                     mental disorders due to primary cerebral disease
                     mental disorders due to somatic illness
                     mental disorders due to systemic disease affecting the brain
       Code first the underlying physiological condition
       Excludes 1:   unspecified dementia (F03)
       Excludes 2:   delirium due to known physiological condition (F05)
                       dementia as classified in F01–F02
                       other mental disorders associated with alcohol and psychoactive substances
                         (F10–F19)
       F06.0   Psychotic disorder with hallucinations due to known physiological condition
       F06.1   Catatonic disorder due to known physiological condition
       F06.2   Psychotic disorder with delusions due to known physiological condition
       F06.3   Mood disorder due to known physiological condition
               F06.30   Mood disorder due to known physiological condition, unspecified
               F06.31   Mood disorder due to known physiological condition with depressive features
               F06.32   Mood disorder due to known physiological condition with major depressive-like episode
               F06.33   Mood disorder due to known physiological condition with manic features
               F06.34   Mood disorder due to known physiological condition with mixed features
       F06.4   Anxiety disorder due to known physiological condition
       F06.8   Other specified mental disorders due to known physiological condition
       F06.9   Unspecified mental disorder due to known physiological condition

Each of these codes has an extensive list of *includes* and *excludes* notes to assist the coding professional in selecting the appropriate code. Physicians should be reminded to document the underlying causes in coding these types of conditions.

Chapter 6

Diseases of the Nervous System

Chapter 6 in the ICD-10-CM Tabular List classifies diseases of the nervous system. It includes categories G00 through G99, which are arranged in the following blocks:

G00–G09   Inflammatory diseases of the central nervous system
G10–G13   Systemic atrophies primarily affecting the central nervous system
G20–G26   Extrapyramidal and movement disorders
G30–G32   Other degenerative diseases of the nervous system
G35–G37   Demyelinating diseases of the central nervous system
G40–G47   Episodic and paroxysmal disorders
G50–G59   Nerve, nerve root and plexus disorders
G60–G64   Polyneuropathies and other disorders of the peripheral nervous system
G70–G73   Diseases of myoneural junction and muscle
G80–G83   Cerebral palsy and other paralytic syndromes
G90–G99   Other disorders of the nervous system

Title Changes

A number of block and category title changes have been made in chapter 6 of ICD-10-CM. A few examples of these changes include the following:

ICD-9-CM:	323	Encephalitis, myelitis and encephalomyelitis
ICD-10-CM:	G04	Encephalitis, myelitis and encephalomyelitis
	G05	Encephalitis, myelitis and encephalomyelitis in diseases classified elsewhere

| ICD-9-CM: | 325 | Phlebitis and thrombophlebitis of intracranial venous sinuses |
| ICD-10-CM | G08 | Intracranial and intraspinal phlebitis and thrombophlebitis |

ICD-9-CM:	333	Other extrapyramidal disease and abnormal movement disorders
ICD-10-CM:	G25	Other extrapyramidal and movement disorders
	G26	Extrapyramidal and movement disorders in diseases classified elsewhere

Additions, Deletions, and Combinations

When chapter 6 in ICD-10-CM is compared with chapter 6 of ICD-9-CM, it is evident that many codes have been added, deleted, combined, or moved to another section or chapter. For example, chapter 6 contains a new section titled Intraoperative and postprocedural complications and disorders of nervous system, not elsewhere classified. The section is further divided into four- and five-character codes and reflects those conditions (hemorrhage, hematoma, reactions, puncture or laceration of organs, and so on) that generally are classified to the complications section of ICD-9-CM chapter 17.

Examples of codes that have been moved from one chapter to another include the following:

- In ICD-9-CM, Dana-Putnam syndrome is classified to codes 281.0, Pernicious anemia, and 336.2, Subacute combined degeneration of spinal cord in diseases classified elsewhere, in chapter 4, Diseases of the Blood and Blood-Forming Organs. In ICD-10-CM, the condition is classified to subcategory G32.0 of chapter 6, Diseases of the Nervous System.

- In ICD-9-CM, basilar and carotid artery syndromes, transient global amnesia, and transient cerebral ischemic attack are classified to chapter 7, Diseases of the Circulatory System; in ICD-10-CM, they are classified to G45, Transient cerebral ischemic attacks and related syndromes, in chapter 6.

Examples of codes that have been moved from one section to another include the following:

- In ICD-9-CM, cataplexy and narcolepsy are assigned a separate category code (347); in ICD-10-CM, these conditions are grouped in code G47.4 under category G47, Organic sleep disorders.

- In ICD-9-CM, Reye's syndrome (331.81) is grouped to 331.8, Other cerebral degenerations; in ICD-10-CM, this condition is coded G93.7 (G93, Other disorders of the brain).

These types of changes should not be a problem for the coding professional because the Alphabetic Index provides directions to the correct codes and chapters.

Finally, sections 360 through 379, Disorders of the Eye and Adnexa, and 380 through 389, Diseases of the Ear and Mastoid Process, in chapter 6 of ICD-9-CM have been reclassified as chapters 7 and 8, respectively, in ICD-10-CM.

Expansions

A number of codes for diseases of the nervous system have been expanded in ICD-10-CM.

Alzheimer's Disease

The category for Alzheimer's disease (G30) has been expanded in ICD-10-CM to reflect onset (early versus late). In addition, a note directs users to assign an additional code for any associated behavioral disturbance (F02.–) or delirium (F05). For example:

ICD-9-CM:	331.0	Alzheimer's disease
ICD-10-CM:	G30	Alzheimer's disease
	G30.0	Alzheimer's disease with early onset
	G30.1	Alzheimer's disease with late onset
	G30.8	Other Alzheimer's disease
	G30.9	Alzheimer's disease, unspecified

Migraine

The code for migraine (G43) has been expanded to fifth characters that indicate the presence or absence of status migrainosus. In addition, the terminology used to describe the types of migraines has been changed. For example:

ICD-9-CM: 346   Migraine
ICD-10-CM: G43   Migraine
          G43.0   Migraine without aura [common migraine]
               G43.00   Migraine without aura, without status migrainosus
               G43.01   Migraine without aura, with status migrainosus
          G43.1   Migraine with aura [classical migraine]
               G43.10   Migraine with aura, without status migrainosus
               G43.11   Migraine with aura, with status migrainosus
          G43.3   Complicated migraine
          G43.8   Other migraine
          G43.9   Migraine, unspecified

Inflammatory and Toxic Neuropathy

ICD-9-CM category 357, Inflammatory and toxic neuropathy, has been split into five categories in ICD-10-CM: G61, Inflammatory polyneuropathy; G62, Other and unspecified polyneuropathies; G63, Polyneuropathy in diseases classified elsewhere; G64, Other disorders of peripheral nervous system; and G65, Sequelae of inflammatory and toxic polyneuropathies.

Expansions to Category Codes

In numerous instances, codes included as subcategory codes in ICD-9-CM have been given a specific category code in ICD-10-CM and expanded at the fourth- or fifth-character level. Changes in these categories should be conveyed to all physicians to make them fully aware of the documentation changes needed for accurate coding. For example:

ICD-9-CM: 332.1   Secondary Parkinsonism
ICD-10-CM: G21   Secondary parkinsonism
          G21.0   Malignant neuroleptic syndrome
          G21.1   Other drug-induced secondary parkinsonism
          G21.2   Secondary parkinsonism due to other external agents
          G21.3   Postencephalitic parkinsonism
          G21.8   Other secondary parkinsonism
          G21.9   Secondary parkinsonism, unspecified

ICD-9-CM: 333.6   Idiopathic torsion dystonia
ICD-10-CM: G24   Dystonia
          G24.0   Drug-induced dystonia
               G24.00   Drug-induced dystonia, unspecified
               G24.01   Drug-induced acute dystonia
               G24.02   Drug-induced tardive dyskinesia
               G24.09   Other drug-induced dystonia
          G24.1   Idiopathic familial dystonia
          G24.2   Idiopathic nonfamilial dystonia
          G24.3   Spasmodic torticollis
          G24.4   Idiopathic orofacial dystonia
          G24.5   Blepharospasm
          G24.8   Other dystonia
          G24.9   Dystonia, unspecified

ICD-9-CM: 358.0   Myasthenia gravis
ICD-10-CM: G70   Myasthenia gravis and other myoneural disorders
                      G70.0   Myasthenia gravis
                                G70.00   Myasthenia gravis without (acute) exacerbation
                                G70.01   Myasthenia gravis with (acute) exacerbation
                      G70.1   Toxic myoneural disorders
                      G70.2   Congenital and developmental myasthenia
                      G70.8   Other specified myoneural disorders
                      G70.9   Myoneural disorder, unspecified

In general, chapter 6 of ICD-10-CM contains a greater degree of specificity for many of the listed codes. Because of this, expansion into fourth and fifth characters is common throughout.

Expansions to Include Notes

Some of the codes in chapter 6 of ICD-10-CM have been expanded to include notes that give instructions to (1) use an additional external cause code to identify causation, (2) code first underlying neoplasm (C00–D48), or (3) code first underlying disease. Examples include:

G02   Meningitis in other infectious and parasitic diseases classified elsewhere
           Code first underlying disease, such as:
                poliovirus infection (A80.–)

G13.0   Paraneoplastic neuromyopathy and neuropathy
           Carcinomatous neuromyopathy
           Sensorial paraneoplastic neuropathy [Denny Brown]
           Code first underlying neoplasm (C00–D48)

G62.82 Radiation-induced polyneuropathy
           Use additional external cause code (W88–W90, X39.0–) to identify cause

Changes in Terminology

A number of category code revisions have been made throughout chapter 6 to better reflect the contents of a category or a change in terminology. For example, users should note a change in terminology with regard to epilepsy. The descriptions of some of the types of epilepsy have been changed between ICD-9-CM category 345 and ICD-10-CM category G40. Category G40 includes the following:

G40   Epilepsy and seizures
      G40.0   Localization-related (focal) (partial) idiopathic epilepsy and epileptic syndromes with seizures of localized onset
            G40.00   Localization-related (focal) (partial) idiopathic epilepsy and epileptic syndromes with seizures of localized onset, not intractable
                  G40.001   Localization-related (focal) (partial) idiopathic epilepsy and epileptic syndromes with seizures of localized onset, not intractable, with status epilepticus
                  G40.009   Localization-related (focal) (partial) idiopathic epilepsy and epileptic syndromes with seizures of localized onset, not intractable, without status epilepticus

G40.01　Localization-related (focal) (partial) idiopathic epilepsy and epileptic syndromes with seizures of localized onset, intractable

　　　　G40.011　Localization-related (focal) (partial) idiopathic epilepsy and epileptic syndromes with seizures of localized onset, intractable, with status epilepticus

　　　　G40.019　Localization-related (focal) (partial) idiopathic epilepsy and epileptic syndromes with seizures of localized onset, intractable, without status epilepticus

G40.1　Localization-related (focal) (partial) symptomatic epilepsy and epileptic syndromes with simple partial seizures

　　　G40.10　Localization-related (focal) (partial) symptomatic epilepsy and epileptic syndromes with simple partial seizures, not intractable

　　　　　G40.101　Localization-related (focal) (partial) symptomatic epilepsy and epileptic syndromes with simple partial seizures, not intractable, with status epilepticus

　　　　　G40.109　Localization-related (focal) (partial) symptomatic epilepsy and epileptic syndromes with simple partial seizures, not intractable, without status epilepticus

　　　G40.11　Localization-related (focal) (partial) symptomatic epilepsy and epileptic syndromes with simple partial seizures, intractable

　　　　　G40.111　Localization-related (focal) (partial) symptomatic epilepsy and epileptic syndromes with simple partial seizures, intractable, with status epilepticus

　　　　　G40.119　Localization-related (focal) (partial) symptomatic epilepsy and epileptic syndromes with simple partial seizures, intractable, without status epilepticus

G40.2　Localization-related (focal) (partial) symptomatic epilepsy and epileptic syndromes with complex partial seizures

　　　G40.20　Localization-related (focal) (partial) symptomatic epilepsy and epileptic syndromes with complex partial seizures, not intractable

　　　　　G40.201　Localization-related (focal) (partial) symptomatic epilepsy and epileptic syndromes with complex partial seizures, not intractable, with status epilepticus

　　　　　G40.209　Localization-related (focal) (partial) symptomatic epilepsy and epileptic syndromes with complex partial seizures, not intractable, without status epilepticus

　　　G40.21　Localization-related (focal) (partial) symptomatic epilepsy and epileptic syndromes with complex partial seizures, intractable

　　　　　G40.211　Localization-related (focal) (partial) symptomatic epilepsy and epileptic syndromes with complex partial seizures, intractable, with status epilepticus

　　　　　G40.219　Localization-related (focal) (partial) symptomatic epilepsy and epileptic syndromes with complex partial seizures, intractable, without status epilepticus

G40.3　Generalized idiopathic epilepsy and epileptic syndromes

　　　G40.30　Generalized idiopathic epilepsy and epileptic syndromes, not intractable

　　　　　G40.301　Generalized idiopathic epilepsy and epileptic syndromes, not intractable, with status epilepticus

　　　　　G40.309　Generalized idiopathic epilepsy and epileptic, not intractable, without status epilepticus

　　　G40.31　Generalized idiopathic epilepsy and epileptic syndromes, intractable

　　　　　G40.311　Generalized idiopathic epilepsy and epileptic syndromes, intractable, with status epilepticus

　　　　　G40.319　Generalized idiopathic epilepsy and epileptic, intractable, without status epilepticus

G40.4 Other generalized epilepsy and epileptic syndromes
    G40.40 Other generalized epilepsy and epileptic syndromes, not intractable
        G40.401 Other generalized epilepsy and epileptic syndromes, not intractable, with status epilepticus
        G40.409 Other generalized epilepsy and epileptic syndromes, not intractable, without status epilepticus
    G40.41 Other generalized epilepsy and epileptic syndromes, intractable
        G40.401 Other generalized epilepsy and epileptic syndromes, intractable, with status epilepticus
        G40.409 Other generalized epilepsy and epileptic syndromes, intractable, without status epilepticus
G40.5 Special epileptic syndromes
    G40.50 Special epileptic syndromes, not intractable
        G40.501 Special epileptic syndromes, not intractable, with status epilepticus
        G40.509 Special epileptic syndromes, not intractable, without status epilepticus
    G40.51 Special epileptic syndromes, intractable
        G40.511 Special epileptic syndromes, intractable, with status epilepticus
        G40.519 Special epileptic syndromes, intractable, without status epilepticus
G40.8 Other epilepsy and seizures
    G40.80 Other epilepsy, not intractable
        G40.801 Other epilepsy, not intractable, with status epilepticus
        G40.809 Other epilepsy, not intractable, without status epilepticus
    G40.81 Other epilepsy, intractable
        G40.811 Other epilepsy, intractable, with status epilepticus
        G30.819 Other epilepsy, intractable, without status epilepticus
G40.9 Epilepsy, unspecified
    G40.90 Epilepsy, unspecified, not intractable
        G40.901 Epilepsy, unspecified, not intractable, with status epilepticus
        G40.909 Epilepsy, unspecified, not intractable, without status epilepticus
    G40.91 Epilepsy, unspecified, intractable
        G40.911 Epilepsy, unspecified, intractable, with status epilepticus
        G40.919 Epilepsy, unspecified, intractable, without status epilepticus

Physicians should be made aware of these changes and asked to use the terminology as reflected in ICD-10-CM.

Another example of terminology changes is reflected in the codes for mononeuropathies of the upper and lower limbs (G56 and G57). The new terminology specifies right side, left side, and unspecified side for each listed condition. For example:

ICD-9-CM: 354.0 Carpal tunnel syndrome
ICD-10-CM: G56.0 Carpal tunnel syndrome
        G56.00 Carpal tunnel syndrome, unspecified side
        G56.01 Carpal tunnel syndrome, right side
        G56.02 Carpal tunnel syndrome, left side

Chapter 7

Diseases of the Eye and Adnexa

Chapter 7 in the ICD-10-CM Tabular List classifies diseases of the eye and adnexa. It includes categories H00 through H59, which are grouped in the following blocks:

H00–H05   Disorders of eyelid, lacrimal system and orbit
H10–H13   Disorders of the conjunctiva
H15–H21   Disorders of sclera, cornea, iris and ciliary body
H25–H28   Disorders of lens
H30–H36   Disorders of choroid and retina
H40–H42   Glaucoma
H43–H45   Disorders of vitreous body and globe
H46–H47   Disorders of optic nerve and visual pathways
H49–H52   Disorders of ocular muscles, binocular movement, accommodation and refraction
H53–H54   Visual disturbances and blindness
H55–H59   Others disorders of eye and adnexa

This is an entirely new chapter in ICD-10-CM. In ICD-9-CM, the conditions discussed in this chapter are located in chapter 6, Diseases of the Nervous System and Sense Organs. However, very few major changes have been made in the content of the codes.

Title Changes

In ICD-10-CM, changes have been made in the titles of codes to better reflect their intent. For example:

ICD-9-CM: 374.55   Hypotrichosis of eyelid
ICD-10-CM: H02.72 Madarosis of eyelid and periocular area

Additions, Deletions, and Combinations

When chapter 7 of ICD-10-CM is compared with chapter 6 of ICD-9-CM, it is evident that some codes have been added, deleted, combined, or moved to another section or chapter. In some cases, new category codes for conditions that did not have a specific code in ICD-9-CM have been added. For example:

H10.51   Ligneous conjunctivitis

H11.01   Amyloid pterygium

H16.26   Vernal keratoconjunctivitis, with limbar and corneal involvement

H21.33   Parasitic cyst of iris, ciliary body or anterior chamber

In some cases, codes have been rearranged. For example, in ICD-10-CM, code H16.24, Ophthalmia nodosa, is located in categories H15 through H21, Disorders of the sclera, cornea, iris and ciliary body. In ICD-9-CM, this condition is included under category 360, Disorders of the globe.

Expansions

Although the codes have not changed, most have been expanded to the fourth-, fifth-, or sixth-character primarily to show the specific anatomy and laterality of the structures. For example:

H00   Hordeolum and chalazion
    H00.0   Hordeolum (externum) (internum) of eyelid
        H00.01   Hordeolum externum
            H00.011   Hordeolum externum right upper eyelid
            H00.012   Hordeolum externum right lower eyelid
            H00.013   Hordeolum externum right eye, unspecified eyelid
            H00.014   Hordeolum externum left upper eyelid
            H00.015   Hordeolum externum left lower eyelid
            H00.016   Hordeolum externum left eye, unspecified eyelid
            H00.019   Hordeolum externum unspecified eye, unspecified eyelid
H20   Iridocyclitis
    H20.0   Acute and subacute iridocyclitis
        H20.00   Unspecified acute and subacute iridocyclitis
        H20.01   Primary iridocyclitis
            H20.011   Primary iridocyclitis, right eye
            H20.012   Primary iridocyclitis, left eye
            H20.013   Primary iridocyclitis, bilateral
            H20.019   Primary iridocyclitis, unspecified eye

Forms and documentation should reflect, whenever possible, the exact site of the ocular condition.

Changes in Terminology

The term *senile cataract* used in ICD-9-CM is not used in the titles of the codes in ICD-10-CM; instead, the term *age-related cataract* is used. For example:

H25   Age-related cataract
    Senile cataract
    H25.0   Age-related incipient cataract
    H25.1   Age-related nuclear cataract
    H25.2   Age-related cataract, morgagnian type
    H25.8   Other age-related cataract
    H25.9   Unspecified age-related cataract

Laterality is reflected at the fifth- or sixth-character level for these codes. For example:

H25.1   Age-related nuclear cataract
    H25.10   Age-related nuclear cataract, unspecified eye
    H25.11   Age-related nuclear cataract, right eye
    H25.12   Age-related nuclear cataract, left eye
    H25.13   Age-related nuclear cataract, bilateral

Changes in Structure

Several categories throughout ICD-10-CM chapter 7 relate to eye disorders in diseases classified elsewhere. For example:

H28   Cataract in diseases classified elsewhere
    Code first underlying disease, such as:
        hypoparathyroidism (E20.–)
        myotonia (G71.1)
        myxedema (E03.–)
        protein-calorie malnutrition (E40–E46)
    Excludes 1:   cataract in diabetes mellitus (E08.33, E09.33, E10.33, E11.33, E13.33, E14.33)

H32   Chorioretinal disorders in diseases classified elsewhere
    Code first underlying disease, such as:
        congenital toxoplasmosis (P37.1)
        histoplasmosis (B39.–)
        leprosy (A30.–)
    Excludes 1:   chorioretinitis (in):
            toxoplasmosis (acquired) (B58.01)
            tuberculosis (A18.53)

H42   Glaucoma in diseases classified elsewhere
    Code first underlying condition, such as:
        amyloidosis (E85)
        aniridia (Q13.1)
        Lowe's syndrome (E72.03)
        Reiger's anomaly (Q13.81)
        specified metabolic disorder (E70–E90)
    Excludes 1:   glaucoma (in):
            diabetes mellitus (E08.39, E09.39, E10.39, E11.39, E13.39, E14.39)
            onchocerciasis (B73.02)
            syphilis (A52.71)
            tuberculous (A18.59)

Chapter 8

Diseases of the Ear and Mastoid Process

Chapter 8 in the ICD-10-CM Tabular List classifies diseases of the ear and mastoid process. It includes categories H60 through H95, which are grouped in the following blocks:

H60–H62 Diseases of external ear
H65–H75 Diseases of middle ear and mastoid
H80–H83 Diseases of inner ear
H90–H95 Other disorders of ear

This chapter is new, and it is includes conditions that are classified to chapter 6, Diseases of the Nervous System and Sense Organs, in ICD-9-CM.

Title Changes

A number of category and subcategory titles have been changed in the transition of this material from chapter 6 in ICD-9-CM to chapter 8 of ICD-10-CM. A few examples of these changes include the following:

ICD-9-CM: 381   Nonsuppurative otitis media and Eustachian tube disorders
ICD-10-CM: H65   Nonsuppurative otitis media

ICD-9-CM: 385.33   Cholesteatoma of middle ear and mastoid
ICD-10-CM: H71.2   Cholesteatoma of mastoid

ICD-9-CM: 386   Vertiginous syndromes and other disorders of vestibular system
ICD-10-CM: H81   Disorders of vestibular function

ICD-9-CM: 380.10   Infective otitis externa, unspecified
ICD-10-CM: H60.0   Abscess of external ear

Additions, Deletions, and Combinations

When chapter 8 of ICD-10-CM is compared with chapter 6 of ICD-9-CM, it is evident that a number of codes have been added, deleted, combined, or moved. For example:

ICD-9-CM:	381.03	Acute sanguinous otitis media
	381.04	Acute allergic serous otitis media
	381.05	Acute allergic mucoid otitis media
	381.06	Acute allergic sanguinous otitis media
ICD-10-CM:	H65.11	Acute and subacute allergic otitis media (mucoid) (sanguinous) (serous)

    H65.111 Acute and subacute allergic otitis media (mucoid), (sanguinous), (serous), right ear

    H65.112 Acute and subacute allergic otitis media (mucoid), (sanguinous) (serous), left ear

    H65.113 Acute and subacute allergic otitis media (mucoid), (sanguinous) (serous), bilateral

    H65.114 Acute and subacute allergic otitis media (mucoid), (sanguinous) (serous), recurrent right ear

    H65.115 Acute and subacute allergic otitis media (mucoid), (sanguinous) (serous), recurrent, left ear

    H65.116 Acute and subacute allergic otitis media (mucoid), (sanguinous) (serous), recurrent, bilateral

    H65.117 Acute and subacute allergic otitis media (mucoid), (sanguinous) (serous), recurrent, unspecified ear

    H65.119 Acute and subacute allergic otitis media (mucoid), (sanguinous) (serous), unspecified ear

| ICD-9-CM: | Category code(s) in chapter 1, Infectious and Parasitic Diseases |
| ICD-10-CM: | H75 | Other disorders of middle ear and mastoid in diseases classified elsewhere |

    Code first underlying disease

   H75.0 Mastoiditis in infectious and parasitic diseases classified elsewhere

    Excludes 1: mastoiditis (in):
         syphilis (A52.77)
         tuberculosis (A18.03)

    H75.00 Mastoiditis in infectious and parasitic diseases classified elsewhere, unspecified ear

    H75.01 Mastoiditis in infectious and parasitic diseases classified elsewhere, right ear

    H75.02 Mastoiditis in infectious and parasitic diseases classified elsewhere, left ear

    H75.03 Mastoiditis in infectious and parasitic diseases classified elsewhere, bilateral

   H75.8 Other specified disorders of middle ear and mastoid in diseases classified elsewhere

    H75.80 Other specified disorders of middle ear and mastoid in diseases classified elsewhere, unspecified ear

    H75.81 Other specified disorders of right middle ear and mastoid in diseases classified elsewhere

    H75.82 Other specified disorders of left middle ear and mastoid in diseases classified elsewhere

    H75.83 Other specified disorders of middle ear and mastoid in diseases classified elsewhere, bilateral

ICD-9-CM:	380.10	Infective otitits externa, unspecified
ICD-10-CM:	H60.31	Diffuse otitis externa
	H60.32	Hemorrhagic otitis externa

Chapter 8 contains a new section, H95, Intraoperative and postprocedural complications and disorders of ear and mastoid process, not elsewhere classified, which is further divided into four-, five-, and even six-character codes. These codes reflect conditions such as hemorrhage, hematoma, accidental puncture, and stenosis, which would have generally been classified to the complications section of chapter 17 in ICD-9-CM.

Expansions

Although this new chapter in ICD-10-CM basically parallels the corresponding section in ICD-9-CM, there are a number of changes. These changes include greater specificity added at the fourth-, fifth-, and sixth-character levels to most category codes; the delineation of laterality as well as specific sites; and the addition of many more code first underlying disease notes.

Additional examples include the following:

ICD-9-CM:	381.00	Acute nonsuppurative otitis media, unspecified
ICD-10-CM:	H65.1	Other acute nonsuppurative otitis media

    H65.11   Acute and subacute allergic otitis media (mucoid) (sanguinous) (serous)

        H65.111   Acute and subacute allergic otitis media (mucoid) (sanguinous) (serous), right ear

        H65.112   Acute and subacute allergic otitis media (mucoid) (sanguinous) (serous), left ear

        H65.113   Acute and subacute allergic otitis media (mucoid) (sanguinous) (serous), bilateral

        H65.114   Acute and subacute allergic otitis media (mucoid) (sanguinous) (serous), recurrent, right ear

        H65.115   Acute and subacute allergic otitis media (mucoid) (sanguinous) (serous), recurrent, left ear

        H65.116   Acute and subacute allergic otitis media (mucoid) (sanguinous) (serous), recurrent, bilateral

        H65.117   Acute and subacute allergic otitis media (mucoid) (sanguinous) (serous), recurrent, unspecified ear

        H65.119   Acute and subacute allergic otitis media (mucoid) (sanguinous) (serous), unspecified ear

Expansion into Two Category Codes

ICD-9-CM category code 381, Nonsuppurative otitis media and Eustachian tube disorders, is only one of several codes that have been split into two category codes in ICD-10-CM: H65, Nonsuppurative otitis media, and H68, Eustachian salpingitis and obstruction.

Perforation of Tympanic Membrane

ICD-9-CM category code 384.2, Perforation of tympanic membrane, is assigned to category code H72, Perforation of tympanic membrane, in ICD-10-CM. This category now has instructions to code first any associated otitis media (H65.–, H66.1–, H66.2–, H66.3–, H66.4–, H66.9–, and H67.–). Other category and subcategory codes have added notes to code first underlying disease, such as codes H62.4, H75, and H82.

Tympanosclerosis

Coding professionals should note the following change in fifth characters in ICD-10-CM with regard to code 385.0, Tympanosclerosis:

ICD-9-CM: 385.0   Tympanosclerosis

                  385.00   Tympanosclerosis, unspecified as to involvement

                  385.01   Tympanosclerosis involving tympanic membrane only

                  385.02   Tympanosclerosis involving tympanic membrane and ear ossicles

                  385.03   Tympanosclerosis involving tympanic membrane, ear ossicles, and middle ear

                  385.09   Tympanosclerosis involving other combination of structures

ICD-10-CM: H74.0   Tympanosclerosis

                  H74.01   Tympanosclerosis, right ear

                  H74.02   Tympanosclerosis, left ear

                  H74.03   Tympanosclerosis, bilateral

                  H74.09   Tympanosclerosis, unspecified ear

Chapter 9

Diseases of the Circulatory System

Chapter 9 in the ICD-10-CM Tabular List classifies diseases of the circulatory system. It includes categories I00 through I99, which are grouped in the following blocks:

I00–I02   Acute rheumatic fever
I05–I09   Chronic rheumatic heart diseases
I10–I15   Hypertensive diseases
I20–I25   Ischemic heart diseases
I26–I28   Pulmonary heart disease and diseases of pulmonary circulation
I30–I52   Other forms of heart disease
I60–I69   Cerebrovascular diseases
I70–I79   Diseases of arteries, arterioles and capillaries
I80–I89   Diseases of veins, lymphatic vessels and lymph nodes, not elsewhere classified
I95–I99   Other and unspecified disorders of the circulatory system

Title Changes

A number of block and category title changes have been made in chapter 9 of ICD-10-CM. A few examples of these changes include the following:

ICD-9-CM: 430   Subarachnoid hemorrhage
ICD-10-CM: I60   Nontraumatic subarachnoid hemorrhage

ICD-9-CM: 434   Occlusion of cerebral arteries
ICD-10-CM: I66   Occlusion and stenosis of cerebral arteries, not resulting in cerebral infarction

ICD-9-CM: 438   Late effects of cerebrovascular disease
ICD-10-CM: I69   Sequelae of cerebrovascular disease

ICD-9-CM: Diseases of Pulmonary Circulation (415–417)
ICD-10-CM: Pulmonary heart disease and diseases of pulmonary circulation (I26–I28)

Additions, Deletions, and Combinations

When chapter 9 of ICD-10-CM is compared with chapter 7 of ICD-9-CM, it is evident that many codes have been added, deleted, combined, or moved to another section or chapter. For example, Binswanger's disease in chapter 5, Mental Disorders, in ICD-9-CM has been moved to chapter 9 in ICD-10-CM and is coded as I67.3.

In addition, the following codes from chapter 4, Diseases of the Blood and Blood-Forming Organs (280–289), have been moved to chapter 9 in ICD-10-CM:

ICD-9-CM:	289.1	Chronic lymphadenitis
	289.2	Nonspecific mesenteric lymphadenitis
	289.8	Other specified diseases of blood and blood-forming organs
	289.9	Unspecified diseases of blood and blood-forming organs
ICD-10-CM:	I88.0	Nonspecific mesenteric lymphadenitis
	I88.1	Chronic lymphadenitis, except mesenteric
	I88.8	Other nonspecific lymphadenitis
	I88.9	Nonspecific lymphadenitis, unspecified

In ICD-9-CM, the code for gangrene (785.4) is classified in chapter 16, Symptoms, Signs and Ill-Defined Conditions. In chapter 9 of ICD-10-CM, it is coded as I96, Gangrene, not elsewhere classified.

Chapter 9 also includes a new section entitled Intraoperative and postprocedural complications and disorders of the circulatory system, not elsewhere classified (I97), which is further divided into four- and five-character codes. These codes reflect conditions such as hemorrhage, hematoma, accidental puncture and laceration, postcardiotomy syndrome, postmastectomy lymphedema syndrome, and postoperative hypertension, all of which would have generally been classified to the complications section of chapter 17 in ICD-9-CM.

Expansions

A number of codes for diseases of the circulatory system have been expanded in ICD-10-CM. For example, code I07, Rheumatic tricuspid valve diseases, has been expanded in ICD-10-CM to reflect the manifestations of the valve diseases.

ICD-9-CM:	397.0	Diseases of tricuspid valve	
ICD-10-CM:	I07	Rheumatic tricuspid valve diseases	
		I07.0	Rheumatic tricuspid stenosis
		I07.1	Rheumatic tricuspid insufficiency
		I07.2	Rheumatic tricuspid stenosis and insufficiency
		I07.8	Other rheumatic tricuspid valve diseases
		I07.9	Rheumatic tricuspid valve disease, unspecified

Nontraumatic Subarachnoid Hemorrhage

Code I60, Nontraumatic subarachnoid hemorrhage, has been expanded to fourth characters to indicate specific sites. For example:

ICD-9-CM:	430	Subarachnoid hemorrhage	
ICD-10-CM:	I60	Nontraumatic subarachnoid hemorrhage	
		I60.0	Nontraumatic subarachnoid hemorrhage from carotid siphon and bifurcation
		I60.1	Nontraumatic subarachnoid hemorrhage from middle cerebral artery
		I60.2	Nontraumatic subarachnoid hemorrhage from anterior communicating artery

I60.3   Nontraumatic subarachnoid hemorrhage from posterior communicating artery

I60.4   Nontraumatic subarachnoid hemorrhage from basilar artery

I60.5   Nontraumatic subarachnoid hemorrhage from vertebral artery

I60.6   Nontraumatic subarachnoid hemorrhage from other intracranial arteries

I60.7   Nontraumatic subarachnoid hemorrhage from intracranial artery, unspecified

I60.8   Other nontraumatic subarachnoid hemorrhage

I60.9   Nontraumatic subarachnoid hemorrhage, unspecified

Late Effects of Cerebrovascular Disease

Code 438, Late effects of cerebrovascular disease, in ICD-9-CM has been restructured in ICD-10-CM with the expansion of all subcategory codes. The expansion is in the form of specifying laterality, changing subcategory titles, making terminology changes, adding sixth characters, and providing greater specificity in general. For example:

ICD-9-CM: 438   Late effects of cerebrovascular disease

    438.0   Cognitive deficits

    438.1   Speech and language deficits

        438.10   Speech and language deficit, unspecified

        438.11   Aphasia

        438.12   Dysphasia

        438.19   Other speech and language deficits

    438.2   Hemiplegia/hemiparesis

        438.20   Hemiplegia affecting unspecified side

        438.21   Hemiplegia affecting dominant side

        438.22   Hemiplegia affecting nondominant side

    438.3   Monoplegia of upper limb

        438.30   Monoplegia of upper limb affecting unspecified side

        438.31   Monoplegia of upper limb affecting dominant side

        438.32   Monoplegia of upper limb affecting nondominant side

    438.4   Monoplegia of lower limb

        438.40   Monoplegia of lower limb affecting unspecified side

        438.41   Monoplegia of lower limb affecting dominant side

        438.42   Monoplegia of lower limb affecting nondominant side

    438.5   Other paralytic syndrome

        Use additional code to identify type of paralytic syndrome, such as:

            locked-in state (344.81)

            quadriplegia (344.00–344.09)

        438.50   Other paralytic syndrome affecting unspecified side

        438.51   Other paralytic syndrome affecting dominant side

        438.52   Other paralytic syndrome affecting nondominant side

        438.53   Other paralytic syndrome, bilateral

    438.6   Alterations of sensations

    438.7   Disturbances of vision

    438.8   Other late effects of cerebrovascular disease

        438.81   Apraxia

        438.82   Dysphagia

        438.83   Facial weakness

        438.84   Ataxia

        438.85   Vertigo

        438.89   Other late effects of cerebrovascular disease

ICD-10-CM: I69 Sequelae of cerebrovascular disease
  I69.0 Sequelae of nontraumatic subarachnoid hemorrhage
    I69.00 Unspecified late effects of nontraumatic subarachnoid hemorrhage
    I69.01 Cognitive deficits following nontraumatic subarachnoid hemorrhage
    I69.02 Speech and language deficits following nontraumatic subarachnoid hemorrhage
      I69.020 Aphasia following nontraumatic subarachnoid hemorrhage
      I69.021 Dysphasia following nontraumatic subarachnoid hemorrhage
      I69.028 Other speech and language deficits following nontraumatic subarachnoid hemorrhage
    I69.03 Monoplegia of upper limb following nontraumatic subarachnoid hemorrhage
      I69.031 Monoplegia of upper limb following nontraumatic subarachnoid hemorrhage affecting right dominant side
      I69.032 Monoplegia of upper limb following nontraumatic subarachnoid hemorrhage affecting left dominant side
      I69.033 Monoplegia of upper limb following nontraumatic subarachnoid hemorrhage affecting right non-dominant side
      I69.034 Monoplegia of upper limb following nontraumatic subarachnoid hemorrhage affecting left non-dominant side
      I69.039 Monoplegia of upper limb following nontraumatic subarachnoid hemorrhage affecting unspecified side
    I69.04 Monoplegia of lower limb following nontraumatic subarachnoid hemorrhage
      I69.041 Monoplegia of lower limb following nontraumatic subarachnoid hemorrhage affecting right dominant side
      I69.042 Monoplegia of lower limb following nontraumatic subarachnoid hemorrhage affecting left dominant side
      I69.043 Monoplegia of lower limb following nontraumatic subarachnoid hemorrhage affecting right non-dominant side
      I69.044 Monoplegia of lower limb following nontraumatic subarachnoid hemorrhage affecting left non-dominant side
      I69.049 Monoplegia of lower limb following nontraumatic subarachnoid hemorrhage affecting unspecified side
    I69.05 Hemiplegia and hemiparesis following nontraumatic subarachnoid hemorrhage
      I69.051 Hemiplegia and hemiparesis following nontraumatic subarachnoid hemorrhage affecting right dominant side

           I69.052   Hemiplegia and hemiparesis following nontraumatic subarachnoid hemorrhage affecting left dominant side

           I69.053   Hemiplegia and hemiparesis following nontraumatic subarachnoid hemorrhage affecting right non-dominant side

           I69.054   Hemiplegia and hemiparesis following nontraumatic subarachnoid hemorrhage affecting left non-dominant side

           I69.059   Hemiplegia and hemiparesis following nontraumatic subarachnoid hemorrhage affecting unspecified side

I69.06   Other paralytic syndrome following nontraumatic subarachnoid hemorrhage

Use additional code to identify type of paralytic syndrome, such as:

    locked-in state (G83.5)

    quadriplegia (G82.39, G82.49, G82.8)

           I69.061   Other paralytic syndrome following nontraumatic subarachnoid hemorrhage affecting right dominant side

           I69.062   Other paralytic syndrome following nontraumatic subarachnoid hemorrhage affecting left dominant side

           I69.063   Other paralytic syndrome following nontraumatic subarachnoid hemorrhage affecting right non-dominant side

           I69.064   Other paralytic syndrome following nontraumatic subarachnoid hemorrhage affecting left non-dominant side

           I69.065   Other paralytic syndrome following nontraumatic subarachnoid hemorrhage, bilateral

           I69.069   Other paralytic syndrome following nontraumatic subarachnoid hemorrhage affecting unspecified side

I69.09   Other late effects of nontraumatic subarachnoid hemorrhage

           I69.090   Apraxia following nontraumatic subarachnoid hemorrhage

           I69.091   Dysphagia following nontraumatic subarachnoid hemorrhage

           I69.092   Facial weakness following nontraumatic subarachnoid hemorrhage

           I69.093   Ataxia following nontraumatic subarachnoid hemorrhage

           I69.098   Other late effects following nontraumatic subarachnoid hemorrhage

Use additional code to identify the sequelae

I69.1   Sequelae of nontraumatic intracerebral hemorrhage

I69.10   Unspecified late effects of nontraumatic intracerebral hemorrhage

I69.11   Cognitive deficits following nontraumatic intracerebral hemorrhage

I69.12   Speech and language deficits following nontraumatic intracerebral hemorrhage

        I69.120   Aphasia following nontraumatic intracerebral hemorrhage

        I69.121   Dysphasia following nontraumatic intracerebral hemorrhage

        I69.128   Other speech and language deficits following nontraumatic intracerebral hemorrhage

I69.13   Monoplegia of upper limb following nontraumatic intracerebral hemorrhage

        I69.131   Monoplegia of upper limb following nontraumatic intracerebral hemorrhage affecting right dominant side

        I69.132   Monoplegia of upper limb following nontraumatic intracerebral hemorrhage affecting left dominant side

        I69.133   Monoplegia of upper limb following nontraumatic intracerebral hemorrhage affecting right non-dominant side

        I69.134   Monoplegia of upper limb following nontraumatic intracerebral hemorrhage affecting left non-dominant side

        I69.139   Monoplegia of upper limb following nontraumatic intracerebral hemorrhage affecting unspecified side

I69.14   Monoplegia of lower limb following nontraumatic intracerebral hemorrhage

        I69.141   Monoplegia of lower limb following nontraumatic intracerebral hemorrhage affecting right dominant side

        I69.142   Monoplegia of lower limb following nontraumatic intracerebral hemorrhage affecting left dominant side

        I69.143   Monoplegia of lower limb following nontraumatic intracerebral hemorrhage affecting right non-dominant side

        I69.144   Monoplegia of lower limb following nontraumatic intracerebral hemorrhage affecting left non-dominant side

        I69.149   Monoplegia of lower limb following nontraumatic intracerebral hemorrhage affecting unspecified side

I69.15   Hemiplegia and hemiparesis following nontraumatic intracerebral hemorrhage

        I69.151   Hemiplegia and hemiparesis following nontraumatic intracerebral hemorrhage affecting right dominant side

        I69.152   Hemiplegia and hemiparesis following nontraumatic intracerebral hemorrhage affecting left dominant side

        I69.153   Hemiplegia and hemiparesis following nontraumatic intracerebral hemorrhage affecting right non-dominant side

I69.154   Hemiplegia and hemiparesis following nontraumatic intracerebral hemorrhage affecting left non-dominant side

I69.159   Hemiplegia and hemiparesis following nontraumatic intracerebral hemorrhage affecting unspecified side

I69.16   Other paralytic syndrome following nontraumatic intracerebral hemorrhage

Use additional code to identify type of paralytic
    syndrome, such as:
      locked-in state (G83.5)
      quadriplegia (G82.39, G82.49, G82.8)

I69.161   Other paralytic syndrome following nontraumatic intracerebral hemorrhage affecting right dominant side

I69.162   Other paralytic syndrome following nontraumatic intracerebral hemorrhage affecting left dominant side

I69.163   Other paralytic syndrome following nontraumatic intracerebral hemorrhage affecting right non-dominant side

I69.164   Other paralytic syndrome following nontraumatic intracerebral hemorrhage affecting left non-dominant side

I69.165   Other paralytic syndrome following nontraumatic intracerebral hemorrhage, bilateral

I69.169   Other paralytic syndrome following nontraumatic intracerebral hemorrhage affecting unspecified site

I69.19   Other late effects of nontraumatic intracerebral hemorrhage

I69.190   Apraxia following nontraumatic intracerebral hemorrhage

I69.191   Dysphagia following nontraumatic intracerebral hemorrhage

I69.192   Facial weakness following nontraumatic intracerebral hemorrhage

I69.193   Ataxia following nontraumatic intracerebral hemorrhage

I69.198   Other late effects of nontraumatic intracerebral hemorrhage

I69.2   Sequelae of other nontraumatic intracranial hemorrhage

I69.20   Unspecified late effects of other nontraumatic intracranial hemorrhage

I69.21   Cognitive deficits following other nontraumatic intracranial hemorrhage

I69.22   Speech and language deficits following other nontraumatic intracranial hemorrhage

I69.220   Aphasia following other nontraumatic intracranial hemorrhage

I69.221   Dysphasia following other nontraumatic intracranial hemorrhage

I69.228   Other speech and language deficits following other nontraumatic intracranial hemorrhage

I69.23 Monoplegia of upper limb following other nontraumatic intracranial hemorrhage
  I69.231 Monoplegia of upper limb following other nontraumatic intracranial hemorrhage affecting right dominant side
  I69.232 Monoplegia of upper limb following other nontraumatic intracranial hemorrhage affecting left dominant side
  I69.233 Monoplegia of upper limb following other nontraumatic intracranial hemorrhage affecting right non-dominant side
  I69.234 Monoplegia of upper limb following other nontraumatic intracranial hemorrhage affecting left non-dominant side
  I69.239 Monoplegia of upper limb following other nontraumatic intracranial hemorrhage affecting unspecified side

I69.24 Monoplegia of lower limb following other nontraumatic intracranial hemorrhage
  I69.241 Monoplegia of lower limb following other nontraumatic intracranial hemorrhage affecting right dominant side
  I69.242 Monoplegia of upper limb following other nontraumatic intracranial hemorrhage affecting left dominant side
  I69.243 Monoplegia of upper limb following other nontraumatic intracranial hemorrhage affecting right non-dominant side
  I69.244 Monoplegia of upper limb following other nontraumatic intracranial hemorrhage affecting left non-dominant side
  I69.249 Monoplegia of upper limb following other nontraumatic intracranial hemorrhage affecting unspecified side

I69.25 Hemiplegia and hemiparesis following other nontraumatic intracranial hemorrhage
  I69.251 Hemiplegia and hemiparesis following other nontraumatic intracranial hemorrhage affecting right dominant side
  I69.252 Hemiplegia and hemiparesis following other nontraumatic intracranial hemorrhage affecting left dominant side
  I69.253 Hemiplegia and hemiparesis following other nontraumatic intracranial hemorrhage affecting right non-dominant side
  I69.254 Hemiplegia and hemiparesis following other nontraumatic intracranial hemorrhage affecting left non-dominant side
  I69.259 Hemiplegia and hemiparesis following other nontraumatic intracranial hemorrhage affecting unspecified side

I69.26 Other paralytic syndrome following other nontraumatic intracranial hemorrhage

Use additional code to identify type of paralytic
syndrome, such as:
    locked-in state (G83.5)
    quadriplegia (G82.39, G82.49, G82.8)

I69.261   Other paralytic syndrome following other nontraumatic intracranial hemorrhage affecting right dominant side

I69.262   Other paralytic syndrome following other nontraumatic intracranial hemorrhage affecting left dominant side

I69.263   Other paralytic syndrome following other nontraumatic intracranial hemorrhage affecting right non-dominant side

I69.264   Other paralytic syndrome following other nontraumatic intracranial hemorrhage affecting left non-dominant side

I69.265   Other paralytic syndrome following other nontraumatic intracranial hemorrhage, bilateral

I69.269   Other paralytic syndrome following other nontraumatic intracranial hemorrhage affecting unspecified side

I69.29   Other late effects of other nontraumatic intracranial hemorrhage

I69.290   Apraxia following other nontraumatic intracranial hemorrhage

I69.291   Dysphagia following other nontraumatic intracranial hemorrhage

I69.292   Facial weakness following other nontraumatic intracranial hemorrhage

I69.293   Ataxia following other nontraumatic intracranial hemorrhage

I69.298   Other late effects of other nontraumatic intracranial hemorrhage

I69.3   Sequelae of cerebral infarction

I69.30   Unspecified late effects of cerebral infarction

I69.31   Cognitive deficits following cerebral infarction

I69.32   Speech and language deficits following cerebral infarction

I69.320   Aphasia following cerebral infarction

I69.321   Dysphasia following cerebral infarction

I69.328   Other speech and language deficits following cerebral infarction

I69.33   Monoplegia of upper limb following cerebral infarction

I69.331   Monoplegia of upper limb following cerebral infarction affecting right dominant side

I69.332   Monoplegia of upper limb following cerebral infarction affecting left dominant side

I69.333   Monoplegia of upper limb following cerebral infarction affecting right non-dominant side

I69.334   Monoplegia of upper limb following cerebral infarction affecting left non-dominant side

I69.339   Monoplegia of upper limb following cerebral infarction affecting unspecified side

I69.34 Monoplegia of lower limb following cerebral infarction

    I69.341 Monoplegia of lower limb following cerebral infarction affecting right dominant side

    I69.342 Monoplegia of lower limb following cerebral infarction affecting left dominant side

    I69.343 Monoplegia of lower limb following cerebral infarction affecting right non-dominant side

    I69.344 Monoplegia of lower limb following cerebral infarction affecting left non-dominant side

    I69.349 Monoplegia of lower limb following cerebral infarction affecting unspecified side

I69.35 Hemiplegia and hemiparesis following cerebral infarction

    I69.351 Hemiplegia and hemiparesis following cerebral infarction affecting right dominant side

    I69.352 Hemiplegia and hemiparesis following cerebral infarction affecting left dominant side

    I69.353 Hemiplegia and hemiparesis following cerebral infarction affecting right non-dominant side

    I69.354 Hemiplegia and hemiparesis following cerebral infarction affecting left non-dominant side

    I69.359 Hemiplegia and hemiparesis following cerebral infarction affecting unspecified side

I69.36 Other paralytic syndrome following cerebral infarction
Use additional code to identify type of paralytic syndrome, such as:
locked-in state (G83.5)
quadriplegia (G82.39, G82.49, G82.8)

    I69.361 Other paralytic syndrome following cerebral infarction affecting right dominant side

    I69.362 Other paralytic syndrome following cerebral infarction affecting left dominant side

    I69.363 Other paralytic syndrome following cerebral infarction affecting right non-dominant side

    I69.364 Other paralytic syndrome following cerebral infarction affecting left non-dominant side

    I69.365 Other paralytic syndrome following cerebral infarction, bilateral

    I69.369 Other paralytic syndrome following cerebral infarction affecting unspecified side

I69.39 Other late effects of cerebral infarction

    I69.390 Apraxia following cerebral infarction

    I69.391 Dysphagia following cerebral infarction

    I69.392 Facial weakness following cerebral infarction

    I69.393 Ataxia following cerebral infarction

    I69.398 Other late effects of cerebral infarction
Use additional code to identify the sequelae

I69.4 Sequelae of stroke, not specified as hemorrhage or infarction

I69.40 Unspecified late effects of stroke, not specified as hemorrhage or infarction

I69.41 Cognitive deficits following stroke, not specified as hemorrhage or infarction

I69.42 Speech and language deficits following stroke, not specified as hemorrhage or infarction

I69.420   Aphasia following stroke, not specified as hemorrhage or infarction

I69.421   Dysphasia following stroke, not specified as hemorrhage or infarction

I69.428   Other speech and language deficits following stroke, not specified as hemorrhage or infarction

I69.43   Monoplegia of upper limb following stroke, not specified as hemorrhage or infarction

I69.431   Monoplegia of upper limb following stroke, not specified as hemorrhage or infarction affecting right dominant side

I69.432   Monoplegia of upper limb following stroke, not specified as hemorrhage or infarction affecting left dominant side

I69.433   Monoplegia of upper limb following stroke, not specified as hemorrhage or infarction affecting right non-dominant side

I69.434   Monoplegia of upper limb following stroke, not specified as hemorrhage or infarction affecting left non-dominant side

I69.439   Monoplegia of upper limb following stroke, not specified as hemorrhage or infarction affecting unspecified side

I69.44   Monoplegia of lower limb following stroke, not specified as hemorrhage or infarction

I69.441   Monoplegia of lower limb following stroke, not specified as hemorrhage or infarction affecting right dominant side

I69.442   Monoplegia of lower limb following stroke, not specified as hemorrhage or infarction affecting left dominant side

I69.443   Monoplegia of lower limb following stroke, not specified as hemorrhage or infarction affecting right non-dominant side

I69.444   Monoplegia of lower limb following stroke, not specified as hemorrhage or infarction affecting left non-dominant side

I69.449   Monoplegia of lower limb following stroke, not specified as hemorrhage or infarction affecting unspecified side

I69.45   Hemiplegia and hemiparesis following stroke, not specified as hemorrhage or infarction

I69.451   Hemiplegia and hemiparesis following stroke, not specified as hemorrhage or infarction affecting right dominant side

I69.452   Hemiplegia and hemiparesis following stroke, not specified as hemorrhage or infarction affecting left dominant side

I69.453   Hemiplegia and hemiparesis following stroke, not specified as hemorrhage or infarction affecting right non-dominant side

       I69.454 Hemiplegia and hemiparesis following stroke, not specified as hemorrhage or infarction affecting left non-dominant side

       I69.459 Hemiplegia and hemiparesis following stroke, not specified as hemorrhage or infarction affecting unspecified side

     I69.46 Other paralytic syndrome following stroke, not specified as hemorrhage or infarction

      Use additional code to identify type of paralytic syndrome, such as:

       locked-in state (G83.5)

       quadriplegia (G82.39, G82.49, G82.8)

       I69.461 Other paralytic syndrome following stroke, not specified as hemorrhage or infarction affecting right dominant side

       I69.462 Other paralytic syndrome following stroke, not specified as hemorrhage or infarction affecting left dominant side

       I69.463 Other paralytic syndrome following stroke, not specified as hemorrhage or infarction affecting right non-dominant side

       I69.464 Other paralytic syndrome following stroke, not specified as hemorrhage or infarction affecting left non-dominant side

       I69.465 Other paralytic syndrome following stroke, not specified as hemorrhage or infarction, bilateral

       I69.469 Other paralytic syndrome following stroke, not specified as hemorrhage or infarction affecting unspecified side

     I69.49 Other late effects of stroke, not specified as hemorrhage or infarction

       I69.490 Apraxia following stroke, not specified as hemorrhage or infarction

       I69.491 Dysphagia following stroke, not specified as hemorrhage or infarction

       I69.492 Facial weakness following stroke, not specified as hemorrhage or infarction

       I69.493 Ataxia following stroke, not specified as hemorrhage or infarction

       I69.498 Other late effects of stroke, not specified as hemorrhage or infarction

   I69.8 Sequelae of other cerebrovascular diseases

     I69.80 Unspecified late effects of other cerebrovascular disease

     I69.81 Cognitive deficits following other cerebrovascular disease

     I69.82 Speech and language deficits following other cerebrovascular disease

       I69.820 Aphasia following other cerebrovascular disease

       I69.821 Dysphasia following other cerebrovascular disease

       I69.828 Other speech and language deficits following other cerebrovascular disease

     I69.83 Monoplegia of upper limb following other cerebrovascular disease

I69.831 Monoplegia of upper limb following other cerebrovascular disease affecting right dominant side

I69.832 Monoplegia of upper limb following other cerebrovascular disease affecting left dominant side

I69.833 Monoplegia of upper limb following other cerebrovascular disease affecting right non-dominant side

I69.834 Monoplegia of upper limb following other cerebrovascular disease affecting left non-dominant side

I69.839 Monoplegia of upper limb following other cerebrovascular disease affecting unspecified side

I69.84 Monoplegia of lower limb following other cerebrovascular disease

I69.841 Monoplegia of lower limb following other cerebrovascular disease affecting right dominant side

I69.842 Monoplegia of lower limb following other cerebrovascular disease affecting left dominant side

I69.843 Monoplegia of lower limb following other cerebrovascular disease affecting right non-dominant side

I69.844 Monoplegia of lower limb following other cerebrovascular disease affecting left non-dominant side

I69.849 Monoplegia of lower limb following other cerebrovascular disease affecting unspecified side

I69.85 Hemiplegia and hemiparesis following other cerebrovascular disease

I69.851 Hemiplegia and hemiparesis following other cerebrovascular disease affecting right dominant side

I69.852 Hemiplegia and hemiparesis following other cerebrovascular disease affecting left dominant side

I69.853 Hemiplegia and hemiparesis following other cerebrovascular disease affecting right non-dominant side

I69.854 Hemiplegia and hemiparesis following other cerebrovascular disease affecting left non-dominant side

I69.859 Hemiplegia and hemiparesis following other cerebrovascular disease affecting unspecified side

I69.86 Other paralytic syndrome following other cerebrovascular disease

Use additional code to identify type of paralytic syndrome, such as:
    locked-in state (G83.5)
    quadriplegia (G82.39, G82.49, G82.8)

I69.861 Other paralytic syndrome following other cerebrovascular disease affecting right dominant side

I69.862 Other paralytic syndrome following other cerebrovascular disease affecting left dominant side

I69.863 Other paralytic syndrome following other cerebrovascular disease affecting right non-dominant side

I69.864 Other paralytic syndrome following other cerebrovascular disease affecting left non-dominant side

I69.865 Other paralytic syndrome following other cerebrovascular disease, bilateral

I69.869 Other paralytic syndrome following other cerebrovascular disease affecting unspecified side

I69.89 Other late effects of other cerebrovascular disease

I69.890 Apraxia following other cerebrovascular disease

I69.891 Dysphagia following other cerebrovascular disease

I69.892 Facial weakness following other cerebrovascular disease

I69.893 Ataxia following other cerebrovascular disease

I69.898 Other late effects of other cerebrovascular disease

 Use additional code to identify the sequelae

I69.9 Sequelae of unspecified cerebrovascular diseases

I69.90 Unspecified late effects of unspecified cerebrovascular disease

I69.91 Cognitive deficits following unspecified cerebrovascular disease

I69.92 Speech and language deficits following unspecified cerebrovascular disease

I69.920 Aphasia following unspecified cerebrovascular disease

I69.921 Dysphasia following unspecified cerebrovascular disease

I69.928 Other speech and language deficits following unspecified cerebrovascular disease

I69.93 Monoplegia of upper limb following unspecified cerebrovascular disease

I69.931 Monoplegia of upper limb following unspecified cerebrovascular disease affecting right dominant side

I69.932 Monoplegia of upper limb following unspecified cerebrovascular disease affecting left dominant side

I69.933 Monoplegia of upper limb following unspecified cerebrovascular disease affecting right non-dominant side

I69.934 Monoplegia of upper limb following unspecified cerebrovascular disease affecting left non-dominant side

I69.939 Monoplegia of upper limb following unspecified cerebrovascular disease affecting unspecified side

I69.94 Monoplegia of lower limb following unspecified cerebrovascular disease

I69.941 Monoplegia of lower limb following unspecified cerebrovascular disease affecting right dominant side

I69.942 Monoplegia of lower limb following unspecified cerebrovascular disease affecting left dominant side

I69.943 Monoplegia of lower limb following unspecified cerebrovascular disease affecting right non-dominant side

I69.944 Monoplegia of lower limb following unspecified cerebrovascular disease affecting left non-dominant side

I69.949 Monoplegia of lower limb following unspecified cerebrovascular disease affecting unspecified side

I69.95 Hemiplegia and hemiparesis following unspecified cerebrovascular disease

I69.951 Hemiplegia and hemiparesis following unspecified cerebrovascular disease affecting right dominant side

I69.952 Hemiplegia and hemiparesis following unspecified cerebrovascular disease affecting left dominant side

I69.953 Hemiplegia and hemiparesis following unspecified cerebrovascular disease affecting right non-dominant side

I69.954 Hemiplegia and hemiparesis following unspecified cerebrovascular disease affecting left non-dominant side

I69.959 Hemiplegia and hemiparesis following unspecified cerebrovascular disease affecting unspecified side

I69.96 Other paralytic syndrome following unspecified cerebrovascular disease

Use additional code to identify type of paralytic syndrome, such as:
locked-in state (G83.5)
quadriplegia (G82.39, G82.49, G82.8)

I69.961 Other paralytic syndrome following unspecified cerebrovascular disease affecting right dominant side

I69.962 Other paralytic syndrome following unspecified cerebrovascular disease affecting left dominant side

I69.963 Other paralytic syndrome following unspecified cerebrovascular disease affecting right non-dominant side

I69.964 Other paralytic syndrome following unspecified cerebrovascular disease affecting left non-dominant side

I69.965 Other paralytic syndrome following unspecified cerebrovascular disease, bilateral

I69.969 Other paralytic syndrome following unspecified cerebrovascular disease affecting unspecified side

I69.99 Other late effects of unspecified cerebrovascular disease

I69.990 Apraxia following unspecified cerebrovascular disease

I69.991 Dysphagia following unspecified cerebrovascular disease

I69.992 Facial weakness following unspecified cerebrovascular disease

I69.993 Ataxia following unspecified cerebrovascular disease

I69.998 Other late effects following unspecified cerebrovascular disease
Use additional code to identify the sequelae

Subcategory Codes Expanded to Fifth- and Sixth-Character Levels

In numerous instances, codes included as subcategory codes in ICD-9-CM have been given a specific subcategory code in ICD-10-CM and expanded to the fifth- or sixth-character level. For example:

ICD-9-CM: 440.24 Atherosclerosis of the extremities with gangrene
ICD-10-CM: I70.26 Atherosclerosis of native arteries of extremities with gangrene

I70.261 Atherosclerosis of native arteries of extremities with gangrene, right leg

I70.262 Atherosclerosis of native arteries of extremities with gangrene, left leg

I70.263 Atherosclerosis of native arteries of extremities with gangrene, bilateral legs

I70.268 Atherosclerosis of native arteries of extremities with gangrene, other extremity

I70.269 Atherosclerosis of native arteries of extremities with gangrene, unspecified extremity

Changes in these categories should be conveyed to physicians to make them aware of the documentation needed for accurate coding.

Changes in Instructions and Notes

ICD-10-CM category code I26, Pulmonary embolism, includes instructions to code first pulmonary embolism complicating abortion of ectopic or molar pregnancy (O00–O07, O08.2) and pregnancy, childbirth, and the puerperium (O88.–).

Other subcategory codes have similar notes, for example:

I30.1 Infective pericarditis
Use additional code (B95–B97) to identify infectious agent

I32   Pericarditis in diseases classified elsewhere
        Code first underlying disease, such as:
            uremia (N19)

I85   Esophageal varices
        Use additional code to identify:
            alcohol abuse and dependence (F10.–)
            alcohol dependence, in remission (F10.11)

Hypertensive diseases (I10–I15)
    Use additional code to identify:
        exposure to environmental tobacco smoke (Z58.83)
        history of tobacco use (Z86.43)
        occupational exposure to environmental tobacco smoke (Z57.31)
        tobacco dependence (F17.–)
        tobacco use (Z72.0)

Changes in Terminology

The terminology used to describe several cardiovascular conditions in ICD-10-CM is different than the terms used in ICD-9-CM.

Angina Pectoris

For angina pectoris, the terminology changes are as follows:

ICD-9-CM: 411.1   Intermediate coronary syndrome
ICD-10-CM: I20.0   Unstable angina

ICD-9-CM: 413.1   Prinzmetal angina
ICD-10-CM: I20.1   Angina pectoris with documented spasm

Myocardial Infarction

For acute myocardial infarction, the terminology changes are as follows:

ICD-9-CM: 410   Acute myocardial infarction
                   410.0   Of anterolateral wall
                   410.1   Of other anterior wall
                   410.2   Of inferolateral wall
                   410.3   Of inferoposterior wall
                   410.4   Of other inferior wall
                   410.5   Of other lateral wall
                   410.6   True posterior wall infarction
                   410.7   Subendocardial infarction
                   410.8   Of other specified sites
                   410.9   Unspecified site
ICD-10-CM: I21   Acute myocardial infarction
                   I21.0   Acute transmural myocardial infarction of anterior wall
                   I21.1   Acute transmural myocardial infarction of inferior wall
                   I21.2   Acute transmural myocardial infarction of other sites
                   I21.3   Acute transmural myocardial infarction of unspecified site
                   I21.4   Acute subendocardial myocardial infarction
                   I21.9   Acute myocardial infarction, unspecified

Similar fifth characters apply category I22, Subsequent acute myocardial infarction.

Atherosclerosis

Fifth characters in ICD-9-CM refer to the type of vessel and whether the bypass is native or a graft. The terminology changes are as follows:

ICD-9-CM: 414.0   Coronary atherosclerosis
ICD-10-CM: I25.1   Atherosclerotic heart disease of native coronary artery

Fifth characters in ICD-10-CM refer to whether the atheroslerotic heart disease is without angina, with unspecified angina pectoris, with unstable angina, with angina pectoris documented spasm, or with other forms of angina pectoris.

A separate subcategory, I25.7, deals with bypass graft(s) or coronary artery of a transplanted heart (which closely parallel the fifth digits under category 414 in ICD-9-CM) with added sixth characters specifying the type of angina pectoris.

Pulmonary Embolism

Physicians must specify whether acute cor pulmonale is associated with a pulmonary embolism to support accurate ICD-10-CM coding.

ICD-9-CM: 415.0   Acute cor pulmonale
               415.1   Pulmonary embolism and infarction
ICD-10-CM: I26   Pulmonary embolism
                   I26.0   Pulmonary embolism with acute cor pulmonale
                   I26.9   Pulmonary embolism without acute cor pulmonale

Cardiac Arrest

Physician documentation must specify the underlying cause of the cardiac arrest to support ICD-10-CM code assignment.

ICD-9-CM: 427.5   Cardiac arrest
ICD-10-CM: I46   Cardiac arrest
                   I46.2   Cardiac arrest due to underlying cardiac condition
                   I46.8   Cardiac arrest due to other underlying condition
                   I46.9   Cardiac arrest, cause unspecified

Nontraumatic Subarachnoid Hemorrhage

The section on nontraumatic subarachnoid hemorrhages has been expanded at the fourth-character level to identify the specific artery causing the hemorrhage.

ICD-9-CM: 430   Subarachnoid hemorrhage
ICD-10-CM: I60   Nontraumatic subarachnoid hemorrhage

Myocardial Infarction

Category 410, Acute myocardial infarction, in ICD-9-CM has been subdivided in ICD-10-CM into three categories: I21, Acute myocardial infarction; I22, Subsequent acute myocardial infarction; and I23, Certain current complications following acute myocardial infarction (within the 28-day period). A note under category I23 indicates that a code from category I23 must be used in conjunction with a code from category I21 or I22. The code from category I23 should be sequenced first when it is the reason for encounter or sequenced after the code from category I21 or I22 when the complication of the myocardial infarction (MI) occurs during the encounter for the MI.

In ICD-9-CM, the specific codes that delineate the type of hypertension (malignant, benign, or unspecified) have been deleted in ICD-10-CM. Hypertension no longer uses type as an axis of classification. For example:

ICD-9-CM:	401.0	Essential hypertension, malignant
	401.1	Essential hypertension, benign
	401.9	Essential hypertension, unspecified
ICD-10-CM:	I10	Essential (primary) hypertension

Chapter 10

Diseases of the Respiratory System

Chapter 10 in the ICD-10-CM Tabular List classifies diseases of the respiratory system. It includes categories J00 through J99, which are arranged in the following blocks:

J00–J06	Acute upper respiratory infections
J10–J18	Influenza and pneumonia
J20–J22	Other acute lower respiratory infections
J30–J39	Other diseases of upper respiratory tract
J40–J47	Chronic lower respiratory diseases
J60–J70	Lung diseases due to external agents
J80–J84	Other respiratory diseases principally affecting the interstitium
J85–J86	Suppurative and necrotic conditions of the lower respiratory tract
J90–J94	Other diseases of the pleura
J95–J99	Other diseases of the respiratory system

Title Changes

A number of block and category title changes have been made in chapter 10 of ICD-10-CM. A few examples of category title changes include the following:

ICD-9-CM:	478	Other diseases of upper respiratory tract
ICD-10-CM:	J38	Diseases of vocal cords and larynx, not elsewhere classified
ICD-9-CM:	495	Extrinsic allergic alveolitis
ICD-10-CM:	J67	Hypersensitivity pneumonitis due to organic dust

A few of the block title changes include the following:

ICD-9-CM:	Chronic Obstructive Pulmonary Diseases and Allied Conditions (490–496)
ICD-10-CM:	Chronic lower respiratory diseases (J40–J47)
ICD-9-CM:	Pneumoconioses and Other Lung Diseases Due to External Agents (500–508)
ICD-10-CM:	Lung diseases due to external agents (J60–J70)

Additions, Deletions, and Combinations

When chapter 10 of ICD-10-CM is compared with chapter 8 of ICD-9-CM, it is evident that many codes have been added, deleted, combined, or moved to another section or chapter. For example, chapter 10 of ICD-10-CM contains a new section, Intraoperative and postprocedural complications and disorders of the respiratory system, not elsewhere classified (J95), which is further divided into fourth and fifth characters. Fourth characters describe complications following surgery and postprocedural conditions such as hemorrhage, hematoma, accidental puncture, and so on. Fifth characters further specify the listed complication.

In the following example, two subcategory codes in ICD-9-CM are combined into one category code in ICD-10-CM.

ICD-9-CM:	464.3	Acute epiglottitis
	464.4	Croup
ICD-10-CM:	J05	Acute obstructive laryngitis [croup] and epiglottitis

ICD-9-CM does not have a specific code for acute recurrent sinusitis. ICD-10-CM provides the following subcategory codes to classify this condition:

J01.01	Acute recurrent maxillary sinusitis
J01.11	Acute recurrent frontal sinusitis
J01.21	Acute recurrent ethmoidal sinusitis
J01.31	Acute recurrent sphenoidal sinusitis
J01.41	Acute recurrent pansinusitis
J01.81	Other acute recurrent sinusitis
J01.91	Acute recurrent sinusitis, unspecified

Several codes have been moved from one section to another. For example, passive pneumonia is classified under code 514, Pulmonary congestion and hypostasis, in ICD-9-CM. The condition falls under category J18, Pneumonia, unspecified organism, in ICD-10-CM.

In ICD-9-CM, code 481, Pneumococcal pneumonia [Streptococcus pneumoniae pneumonia], lists as an inclusion term *lobar pneumonia;* in ICD-10-CM, Lobar pneumonia, unspecified, is assigned a separate subcategory code (J18.1) under category J18, Pneumonia, unspecified organism.

In numerous instances, codes included as subcategory codes in ICD-9-CM have been given a specific category code in ICD-10-CM. For example:

ICD-9-CM:	491.0	Simple chronic bronchitis
	491.1	Mucopurulent chronic bronchitis
ICD-10-CM:	J41	Simple and mucopurulent chronic bronchitis
ICD-9-CM:	482.2	Pneumonia due to Hemophilus influenzae [H. influenzae]
ICD-10-CM:	J14	Pneumonia due to to Hemophilus influenzae
ICD-9-CM:	491.2	Obstructive chronic bronchitis
ICD-10-CM:	J44	Other chronic obstructive pulmonary disease
ICD-9-CM:	466.1	Acute bronchiolitis
ICD-10-CM:	J21	Acute bronchiolitis

Expansions

A number of codes for diseases of the respiratory system have been expanded in ICD-10-CM.

Expansions to Reflect Manifestations

Code 487.8, Influenza with involvement of gastrointestinal tract, has been expanded in ICD-10-CM to reflect the manifestations of the influenza:

ICD-9-CM:	487.8	Influenza with other manifestations
ICD-10-CM:	J10.8	Influenza with other manifestations
	J10.81	Influenzal gastroenteritis
	J10.89	Influenza with other manifestations
		Influenzal encephalopathy
		Influenzal myocarditis

Another example of expanded manifestations includes the code for acute bronchitis:

ICD-9-CM:	466	Acute bronchitis and bronchiolitis
ICD-10-CM:	J20	Acute bronchitis
	J20.0	Acute bronchitis due to Mycoplasma pneumoniae
	J20.1	Acute bronchitis due to Hemophilus influenzae
	J20.2	Acute bronchitis due to streptococcus
	J20.3	Acute bronchitis due to coxsackievirus
	J20.4	Acute bronchitis due to parainfluenza virus
	J20.5	Acute bronchitis due to respiratory syncytial virus
	J20.6	Acute bronchitis due to rhinovirus
	J20.7	Acute bronchitis due to echovirus
	J20.8	Acute bronchitis due to other specified organisms
	J20.9	Acute bronchitis, unspecified

Acute Tonsillitis

In ICD-10-CM, the code for acute tonsillitis has been expanded at the fourth-character level (to indicate organism) and the fifth-character level (to indicate acute and recurrent). For example:

ICD-9-CM:	463	Acute tonsillitis
ICD-10-CM:	J03	Acute tonsillitis
	J03.0	Streptococcal tonsillitis
	J03.00	Acute streptococcal tonsillitis, unspecified
	J03.01	Acute recurrent streptococcal tonsillitis
	J03.8	Acute tonsillitis due to other specified organisms
	J03.80	Acute tonsillitis due to other specified organisms
	J03.81	Acute recurrent tonsillitis due to other specified organisms
	J03.9	Acute tonsillitis, unspecified
		Follicular tonsillitis (acute)
		Gangrenous tonsillitis (acute)
		Infective tonsillitis (acute)
		Tonsillitis (acute) NOS
		Ulcerative tonsillitis (acute)
	J03.90	Acute tonsillitis, unspecified
	J03.91	Acute recurrent tonsillitis, unspecified

Acute Pharyngitis

In ICD-10-CM, the code for acute pharyngitis has been expanded to capture the causative organism. For example:

ICD-9-CM:	462	Acute pharyngitis
ICD-10-CM:	J02	Acute pharyngitis
	J02.0	Streptococcal pharyngitis
	J02.8	Acute pharyngitis due to other specified organism
	J02.9	Acute pharyngitis, unspecified

Changes in these categories should be conveyed to physicians to make them aware of the documentation needed for accurate coding.

Expansion to Include Notes

Some of the codes in chapter 10 of ICD-10-CM have been expanded to include notes indicating that an additional code should be assigned. Four types of instructional notes are provided: (1) use additional code to identify the infectious agent, (2) use additional code to identify the virus, (3) code first any associated lung abscess, and (4) code first the underlying disease. For example:

J01   Acute sinusitis
     Use additional code (B95–B97) to identify infectious agent

J10   Influenza
     Use additional code to identify the virus (B97.–)

J15   Bacterial pneumonia, not elsewhere classified
     Code first any associated lung abscess (J85.1)

J91   Pleural effusion in conditions classified elsewhere
     Code first underlying disease, such as:
       filariasis (B74.0–B74.9)

Throughout chapter 10 of ICD-10-CM, the following note has been added to many category codes:

Use additional code, where applicable, to identify:
   exposure to environmental tobacco smoke (Z58.83)
   exposure to tobacco smoke in the perinatal period (P96.6)
   history of tobacco use (Z86.43)
   occupational exposure to environmental tobacco smoke (Z57.31)
   tobacco dependence (F17.–)
   tobacco use (Z72.0)

The following represent categories where this note appears:

J31   Chronic rhinitis, nasopharyngitis and pharyngitis
J33   Nasal polyp
J35   Chronic diseases of tonsils and adenoids
J38   Diseases of vocal cords and larynx, not elsewhere classified

J40   Bronchitis, not specified as acute or chronic
J41   Simple and mucopurulent chronic bronchitis
J42   Unspecified chronic bronchitis
J45   Asthma
J47   Bronchiectasis
J98   Other respiratory disorders

Codes J43, Emphysema; J44, Other chronic obstructive pulmonary disease; and J81, Pulmonary edema, do not contain the note regarding exposure to tobacco smoke during the perinatal period.

Changes in Terminology

The coding professional should note a change in terminology with regard to some codes in ICD-10-CM. For example, in ICD-9-CM, fifth digits under category 464, Acute laryngitis and tracheitis, refer to whether obstruction was present. In ICD-10-CM, however, category J04, Acute laryngitis and tracheitis, refers only to acute laryngitis, acute tracheitis, and acute laryngotracheitis at the fourth-character level with no mention of obstruction.

Asthma is another example. In ICD-9-CM, category code 493 refers to asthma, with fourth digits specifying type (extrinsic, intrinsic, chronic obstructive, and unspecified) and fifth digits delineating the presence or absence of status asthmaticus or an acute exacerbation. In ICD-10-CM, category J45, Asthma, has the following subcategories:

J45   Asthma
    J45.2   Mild intermittent asthma
    J45.3   Mild persistent asthma
    J45.4   Moderate persistent asthma
    J45.5   Severe persistent asthma
    J45.9   Other and unspecified asthma

Fifth characters under this category specify whether the asthma was uncomplicated, with (acute) exacerbation, or with status asthmaticus.

Chapter 11

Diseases of the Digestive System

Chapter 11 in the ICD-10-CM Tabular List classifies diseases of the digestive system. It includes categories K00 through K94, which are arranged in the following blocks:

K00–K14   Diseases of oral cavity and salivary glands
K20–K31   Diseases of esophagus, stomach and duodenum
K35–K38   Diseases of appendix
K40–K46   Hernia
K50–K52   Noninfective enteritis and colitis
K55–K63   Other diseases of intestines
K65–K68   Diseases of peritoneum and retroperitoneum
K70–K77   Diseases of liver
K80–K87   Disorders of gallbladder, biliary tract and pancreas
K90–K94   Other diseases of the digestive system

Title Changes

A number of block and category title changes have been made in chapter 11 of ICD-10-CM. A few examples of these changes include the following:

ICD-9-CM: Other Diseases of Intestines and Peritoneum (560–569)
ICD-10-CM: Other diseases of intestines (K55–K63)

ICD-9-CM: 536   Disorders of function of stomach
ICD-10-CM: K31   Other diseases of stomach and duodenum

ICD-9-CM: Other Diseases of Digestive System (570–579)
ICD-10-CM: Diseases of liver (K70–K77)

ICD-9-CM: 528   Diseases of the oral soft tissues, excluding lesions specific for gingiva and tongue
ICD-10-CM: K12   Stomatitis and related lesions

ICD-9-CM: 521.03   Dental caries extending into pulp
ICD-10-CM: K02.2   Caries of cementum

Changes in category code titles also have been made to ICD-9-CM code 565, Anal fissure and fistula. Currently, the breakdown of codes is 565.0, Anal fissure, and 565.1, Anal fistula. In ICD-10-CM, the title of the category, Abscess of anal and rectal regions (K61), is more inclusive and is delineated at the fourth-character level with new conditions. For example:

K61   Abscess of anal and rectal regions
     K61.0   Anal abscess
     K61.1   Rectal abscess
     K61.2   Anorectal abscess
     K61.3   Ischiorectal abscess
     K61.4   Intrasphincteric abscess

Additions, Deletions, and Combinations

When chapter 11 of ICD-10-CM is compared with chapter 9 of ICD-9-CM, it is evident that many codes have been added, deleted, combined, or moved to another section or chapter. For example, in ICD-9-CM, code 569.84, Angiodysplasia of intestine (without mention of hemorrhage), is located under the section entitled Other specified disorders of intestine. In chapter 11 of ICD-10-CM, code K55.2, Angiodysplasia of colon, is located under the section on vascular disorders of intestine.

Codes 524, Dentofacial anomalies, including malocclusion, and 526, Diseases of the jaw, in ICD-9-CM have been moved from ICD-9-CM chapter 9, Diseases of the Digestive System, to ICD-10-CM chapter 13, Diseases of the musculoskeletal system and connective tissue.

ICD-9-CM: 524   Dentofacial anomalies, including malocculsion
            526   Diseases of the jaws
ICD-10-CM: M26   Dentofacial anomalies [including malocclusion]
           M27   Other diseases of jaws

An example of a new code in ICD-10-CM is the code for alcoholic hepatitis with ascites.

K70.10   Alcoholic hepatitis without ascites
K70.11   Alcoholic hepatitis with ascites

The developers of ICD-10-CM also restructured some of the disease categories to bring together those groups that are in some way related. For example, chapter 11 of ICD-10-CM contains two new blocks: Diseases of liver (K70–K77) and Disorders of gallbladder, biliary tract and pancreas (K80–K87).

Chapter 11 also contains a new section, Intraoperative and postprocedural complications and disorders of digestive system, not elsewhere classified (K91), which is further divided into fourth and fifth characters. The fourth characters describe complications and conditions following surgery and postprocedural conditions such as hemorrhage, hematoma, accidental puncture, and so on. The fifth characters further specify the listed complication.

Expansions

Category K42, Umbilical hernia, includes fourth characters to indicate whether obstruction and gangrene were present.

ICD-9-CM: 551.1   Umbilical hernia with gangrene
ICD-10-CM: K42   Umbilical hernia
       K42.0   Umbilical hernia with obstruction, without gangrene
       K42.1   Umbilical hernia with gangrene
       K42.9   Umbilical hernia without obstruction or gangrene

Crohn's Disease

ICD-10-CM category K50, Crohn's disease, has been expanded to fourth and fifth characters from ICD-9-CM's code 555.9, Regional enteritis, unspecified site. The expansion at the fourth-character level specifies the site of the Crohn's disease, and the fifth-character expansion indicates whether a complication was present. The specific complications include rectal bleeding, intestinal obstruction, fistula, abscess, and other.

ICD-9-CM: 555.9   Regional enteritis, unspecified site
ICD-10-CM: K50   Crohn's disease [regional enteritis]
      K50.0   Crohn's disease of small intestine
        K50.00   Crohn's disease of small intestine without complications
        K50.01   Crohn's disease of small intestine with complications
          K50.011   Crohn's disease of small intestine with rectal bleeding
          K50.012   Crohn's disease of small intestine with intestinal obstruction
          K50.013   Crohn's disease of small intestine with fistula
          K50.014   Crohn's disease of small intestine with abscess
          K50.018   Crohn's disease of small intestine with other complications
          K50.019   Crohn's disease of small intestine with unspecified complications
      K50.1   Crohn's disease of large intestine
        K50.10   Crohn's disease of large intestine without complications
        K50.11   Crohn's disease of large intestine with complications
          K50.111   Crohn's disease of large intestine with rectal bleeding
          K50.112   Crohn's disease of large intestine with intestinal obstruction
          K50.113   Crohn's disease of large intestine with fistula
          K50.114   Crohn's disease of large intestine with abscess
          K50.118   Crohn's disease of large intestine with other complications
          K50.119   Crohn's disease of large intestine with unspecified complications
      K50.8   Crohn's disease of both small and large intestine
        K50.80   Crohn's disease of both small and large intestine without complications
        K50.81   Crohn's disease of both small and large intestine with complications
          K50.811   Crohn's disease of both small and large intestine with rectal bleeding

K50.812 Crohn's disease of both small and large intestine with intestinal obstruction

K50.813 Crohn's disease of both small and large intestine with fistula

K50.814 Crohn's disease of both small and large intestine with abscess

K50.818 Crohn's disease of both small and large intestine with other complication

K50.819 Crohn's disease of both small and large intestine with unspecified complications

K50.9 Crohn's disease, unspecified

   K50.90 Crohn's disease, unspecified, without complications

   K50.91 Crohn's disease, unspecified, with complications

      K50.911 Crohn's disease, unspecified, with rectal bleeding

      K50.912 Crohn's disease, unspecified, with intestinal obstruction

      K50.913 Crohn's disease, unspecified, with fistula

      K50.914 Crohn's disease, unspecified, with abscess

      K50.918 Crohn's disease, unspecified, with other complications

      K50.919 Crohn's disease, unspecified, with unspecified complications

Changes from Subcategory Codes to Category Codes

Subcategory code 564.1, Irritable bowel syndrome, in ICD-9-CM has been given a specific category code in ICD-10-CM and expanded at the fourth-character level.

ICD-9-CM:	564.1	Irritable bowel syndrome
ICD-10-CM:	K58	Irritable bowel syndrome
	K58.0	Irritable bowel syndrome with diarrhea
	K58.9	Irritable bowel syndrome without diarrhea

Other examples of subcategory codes in ICD-9-CM that have been given a specific category code in ICD-10-CM are as follows:

ICD-9-CM:	520.6	Disturbances in tooth eruption
ICD-10-CM:	K01	Embedded and impacted teeth

ICD-9-CM:	536.8	Dyspepsia and other specified disorders of function of stomach
ICD-10-CM:	K30	Dyspepsia

ICD-9-CM:	571.4	Chronic hepatitis
ICD-10-CM:	K73	Chronic hepatitis, not elsewhere classified

ICD-9-CM category code 521 is assigned two category codes in ICD-10-CM.

ICD-9-CM:	521	Diseases of hard tissues of teeth
ICD-10-CM:	K02	Dental caries
	K03	Other diseases of hard tissues of teeth

Expansion to Include Notes

Notes reminding coders to use additional codes to identify accompanying conditions have been added to many category codes in chapter 11 of ICD-10-CM. For example:

K05   Gingivitis and periodontal diseases
         Use additional code to identify:
             alcohol abuse and dependence (F10.–)
             alcohol dependence, in remission (F10.11)
             exposure to environmental tobacco smoke (Z58.83)
             exposure to tobacco smoke in the perinatal period (P96.6)
             history of tobacco use (Z86.43)
             occupational exposure to environmental tobacco smoke (Z57.31)
             tobacco dependence (F17.–)
             tobacco use (Z72.0)

Other categories where this note appears include K11, Diseases of salivary glands; K12, Stomatitis and related lesions; K13, Other diseases of lip and oral mucosa; and K14, Diseases of tongue. Coding professionals should inform physicians about the additional documentation needed.

Other notes in chapter 11 of ICD-10-CM that indicate that an additional code should be used include: (1) use additional code (chapter 20) to identify external cause, (2) code first underlying disease, such as . . . , (3) use additional code to identify manifestations, such as . . . , and (4) use additional code to specify type of infection, such as. . . . For example:

K06.2   Gingival and edentulous alveolar ridge lesions associated with trauma
            Use additional code (chapter 20) to identify external cause

K23   Disorders of esophagus in diseases classified elsewhere
         Code first underlying disease, such as:
             congenital syphilis (A50.5)

K50   Crohn's disease [regional enteritis]
         Use additional code to identify manifestations, such as:
             pyoderma gangrenosum (L88)

K94.02   Colostomy infection
             Use additional code to specify type of infection, such as:
                 cellulitis of abdominal wall (L03.32)
                 septicemia (A40.–, A41.–)

Ulcers

In ICD-9-CM, the presence or absence of obstruction is used as an axis for classifying ulcers (gastric, duodenal, peptic, or gastrojejunal); in ICD-10-CM, the reference to obstruction has been eliminated. For example:

ICD-9-CM: 531.00   Acute gastric ulcer with hemorrhage without mention of obstruction
                         531.01   Acute gastric ulcer with hemorrhage with obstruction
ICD-10-CM: K25.0   Acute gastric ulcer with hemorrhage

Hernias

In ICD-9-CM, hernias are classified by type (inguinal, femoral, ventral, and so on) with fourth-digit subcategories indicating whether gangrene or obstruction was present. Fifth digits specify whether the type of hernia was unilateral or bilateral and/or recurrent. ICD-10-CM still classifies hernias according to type, but the fourth (and in some cases fifth) characters indicate whether obstruction or gangrene was present as well as the laterality and recurrence status. Moreover, two new category codes are provided in ICD-10-CM: K45, Other abdominal hernia, and K46, Unspecified abdominal hernia.

Diverticula of Intestine

In ICD-9-CM, diverticula of the intestines (562) are classified with fourth digits that indicate site (small intestine versus colon) and fifth digits that indicate whether hemorrhage was present. In ICD-10-CM, code K57, Diverticular disease of intestine, is divided into four- and five-character codes. The fourth characters indicate site (small versus large intestine) and whether perforation and abscess are present. The fifth characters further specify whether there was any associated bleeding. There are minor changes in terminology in this section: *hemorrhage* is referred to as *bleeding*.

Cholelithiasis

In ICD-10-CM, the section on cholelithiasis (K80) has been expanded to incorporate cholangitis.

K80   Cholelithiasis
      K80.0   Calculus of gallbladder with acute cholecystitis
      K80.1   Calculus of gallbladder with other cholecystitis
      K80.2   Calculus of gallbladder without cholecystitis
      K80.3   Calculus of bile duct with cholangitis
      K80.4   Calculus of bile duct with cholecystitis
      K80.5   Calculus of bile duct without cholangitis or cholecystitis
      K80.6   Calculus of gallbladder and bile duct with cholecystitis
      K80.7   Calculus of gallbladder and bile duct without cholecystitis
      K80.8   Other cholelithiasis

Fifth characters under this category further indicate whether obstruction was present and whether the condition was acute or chronic.

Chapter 12

Diseases of the Skin and Subcutaneous Tissue

Chapter 12 in the ICD-10-CM Tabular List classifies diseases of the skin and subcutaneous tissue. It includes categories L00 through L99, which are arranged in the following blocks:

L00–L08   Infections of the skin and subcutaneous tissue
L10–L14   Bullous disorders
L20–L30   Dermatitis and eczema
L40–L45   Papulosquamous disorders
L50–L54   Urticaria and erythema
L55–L59   Radiation-related disorders of the skin and subcutaneous tissue
L60–L75   Disorders of skin appendages
L76   Intraoperative and postprocedural complications of dermatologic procedures
L80–L99   Other disorders of the skin and subcutaneous tissue

Chapter 12 of ICD-10-CM represents a complete restructuring of the classification to bring together groups of diseases that are related to one another in some way. In doing so, greater specificity has been added to almost all codes at either the fourth- or fifth-character level. Chapter 12 of ICD-9-CM includes only the following three subchapters:

Infections of Skin and Subcutaneous Tissue (680–686)
Other Inflammatory Conditions of Skin and Subcutaneous Tissue (690–698)
Other Diseases of Skin and Subcutaneous Tissue (700–709)

These three subchapters in ICD-9-CM have been expanded in ICD-10-CM to create the nine blocks listed above.

Title Changes

A number of block and category title changes have been made in chapter 12 of ICD-9-CM. For example:

ICD-9-CM: 681   Cellulitis and abscess of finger and toe
                        682   Other cellulitis and abscess
ICD-10-CM: L03   Cellulitis and acute lymphangitis

ICD-9-CM: 685   Pilonidal cyst
ICD-10-CM: L05   Pilonidal cyst and sinus

ICD-9-CM: 704.1 Hirsutism
ICD-10-CM: L68   Hypertrichosis

Additions, Deletions, and Combinations

Erythrasma is coded to subcategory code 039.0 in chapter 1, Infectious and Parasitic Diseases, of ICD-9-CM. In ICD-10-CM, the condition is classified to subcategory L08.1, Erythrasma.

Another condition transferred from chapter 1 in ICD-9-CM to chapter 12 in ICD-10-CM is 136.0, Ainhum. In ICD-10-CM, this condition is coded as L94.6.

A new section in chapter 12, Intraoperative and postprocedural complications of dermatologic procedures (L76), is further divided into four- and five-character codes. The fourth characters describe complications and conditions following surgery and postprocedural conditions such as hemorrhage, hematoma, accidental puncture, and so on. The fifth characters further specify the listed complications.

These types of changes should not present a problem for coding professionals and other users of ICD-10-CM because the Alphabetic Index provides directions to the correct codes.

Expansions

A number of codes for diseases of the skin and subcutaneous tissue have been expanded in ICD-10-CM. Although the material in chapter 12 of ICD-10-CM parallels the material in chapter 12 of ICD-9-CM fairly closely as far as specific conditions go, greater specificity is delineated throughout the ICD-10-CM codes at the fourth-, fifth-, and even sixth-character levels.

Subcategory Codes Changed to Category Code

In numerous instances, codes included as subcategory codes in ICD-9-CM have been given a specific category code in ICD-10-CM and expanded at the fourth- or fifth-character level. For example:

ICD-9-CM: 694.4 Pemphigus
ICD-10-CM: L10   Pemphigus
           L10.0   Pemphigus vulgaris
           L10.1   Pemphigus vegetans
           L10.2   Pemphigus foliaceous
           L10.3   Brazilian pemphigus [fogo selvagem]
           L10.4   Pemphigus erythematosus
           L10.5   Drug-induced pemphigus
           L10.8   Other pemphigus
                L10.81   Paraneoplastic pemphigus
                L10.89   Other pemphigus
           L10.9   Pemphigus, unspecified

ICD-9-CM: 704.01 Alopecia areata
ICD-10-CM: L63   Alopecia areata
           L63.0   Alopecia (capitis) totalis
           L63.1   Alopecia universalis
           L63.2   Ophiasis
           L63.8   Other alopecia areata
           L63.9   Alopecia areata, unspecified

```
ICD-9-CM:    694.5   Pemphigoid
ICD-10-CM:   L12     Pemphigoid
                     L12.0   Bullous pemphigoid
                     L12.1   Cicatricial pemphigoid
                     L12.2   Chronic bullous disease of childhood
                     L12.3   Acquired epidermolysis bullosa
                             L12.30   Acquired epidermolysis bullosa, unspecified
                             L12.31   Epidermolysis bullosa due to drug
                             L12.35   Other acquired epidermolysis bullosa
                     L12.8   Other pemphigoid
                     L12.9   Pemphigoid, unspecified
```

Decubitus Ulcer

Code 707.0, Decubitus ulcer, in ICD-9-CM has been greatly expanded in ICD-10-CM with new codes added to further classify this disorder.

```
ICD-9-CM:    707.0   Decubitus ulcer
ICD-10-CM:   L89     Decubitus ulcer
                     L89.0   Decubitus ulcer of back
                             L89.00   Decubitus ulcer of unspecified part of back
                                      L89.001   Decubitus ulcer of unspecified part of back
                                                limited to breakdown of the skin
                                      L89.002   Decubitus ulcer of unspecified part of back
                                                with fat layer exposed
                                      L89.003   Decubitus ulcer of unspecified part of back
                                                with necrosis of muscle
                                      L89.004   Decubitus ulcer of unspecified part of back
                                                with necrosis of bone
                                      L89.009   Decubitus ulcer of unspecified part of back
                                                with unspecified severity
```

At the fourth-character level, additional codes delineate the specific parts of the back and buttock (right upper back, left upper back, right lower back, left lower back, sacral region, buttock, contiguous site of back and buttock, and so on). Fifth characters under each site refer to the breakdown of skin, fat layer exposed, necrosis of muscle or bone, and unspecified severity. The same fifth-character breakdown that applies to category L89 also applies to category L97, Non-decubitus chronic ulcer of lower limb, not elsewhere classified.

Impetigo

ICD-9-CM code for impetigo has been expanded in ICD-10-CM to reflect the specific types of impetigo.

```
ICD-9-CM:    684   Impetigo
ICD-10-CM:   L01   Impetigo
                   L01.0   Impetigo
                           L01.00   Impetigo, unspecified
                           L01.01   Non-bullous impetigo
                           L01.02   Bockhart's impetigo
                           L01.03   Bullous impetigo
                           L01.09   Other impetigo
                   L01.1   Impetiginization of other dermatoses
```

Expansion to Include Notes

Some of the codes in chapter 12 of ICD-10-CM have been expanded to include notes indicating that an additional code should be used: (1) use additional code (B95–B97) to identify the organism, (2) code first (T36–T65) to identify drug or substance, (3) code first underlying disease, and (4) code first any associated condition, as shown below:

Infections of the skin and subcutaneous tissue (L00–L08)
Use additional code (B95–B97) to identify infectious agent

L02   Cutaneous abscess, furuncle and carbuncle
      Use additional code to identify organism (B95–B96)

L23   Allergic contact dermatitis
      Code first (T36–T65) to identify drug or substance

L45   Papulosquamous disorders in diseases classified elsewhere
      Code first underlying disease

L97   Non-decubitus chronic ulcer of lower limb, not elsewhere classified
      Code first any associated underlying condition

Under section L20 through L30, Dermatitis and eczema, a note concerning terminology specific to ICD-10-CM is provided:

Dermatitis and eczema (L20–L30)
Note: In this block the terms dermatitis and eczema are used synonymously and interchangeably.

Psoriasis

Category L40, Psoriasis, has been expanded in ICD-10-CM to reflect the manifestations of psoriasis. For example:

ICD-9-CM:	696.0	Psoriatic arthropathy
	696.1	Other psoriasis
ICD-10-CM:	L40	Psoriasis

L40.0   Psoriasis vulgaris
L40.1   Generalized pustular psoriasis
L40.2   Acrodermatitis continua
L40.3   Pustulosis palmaris et plantaris
L40.4   Guttate psoriasis
L40.5   Arthropathic psoriasis
    L40.50   Arthropathic psoriasis, unspecified
    L40.51   Distal interphalangeal psoriatic arthropathy
    L40.52   Psoriatic arthritis mutilans
    L40.53   Psoriatic spondylitis
    L40.54   Psoriatic juvenile arthropathy
    L40.59   Other psoriatic arthropathy
L40.8   Other psoriasis
L40.9   Psoriasis, unspecified

Chapter 13

Diseases of the Musculoskeletal System and Connective Tissue

Chapter 13 in the ICD-10-CM Tabular List classifies diseases of the musculoskeletal system and connective tissue. It includes categories M00 through M99, which are arranged in the following blocks:

M00–M02   Infectious arthropathies
M05–M14   Inflammatory polyarthropathies
M15–M19   Osteoarthritis
M20–M25   Other joint disorders
M26–M27   Dentofacial anomalies [including malocclusion] and other disorders of jaw
M30–M36   Systemic connective tissue disorders
M40–M43   Deforming dorsopathies
M45–M49   Spondylopathies
M50–M54   Other dorsopathies
M60–M63   Disorders of muscles
M65–M67   Disorders of synovium and tendon
M70–M79   Other soft tissue disorders
M80–M85   Disorders of bone density and structure
M86–M90   Other osteopathies
M91–M94   Chondropathies
M95–M99   Other disorders of the musculoskeletal system and connective tissue

Title Changes

A number of block and category title changes have been made in chapter 13 of ICD-10-CM. A few examples of these changes include the following:

ICD-9-CM: Arthropathies and related disorders (710–719)
ICD-10-CM: Arthropathies (M00–M25)

ICD-9-CM: 714   Rheumatoid arthritis and other inflammatory polyarthropathies
ICD-10-CM: M05   Rheumatoid arthritis with rheumatoid factor

ICD-9-CM: 736   Other acquired deformities of limbs
ICD-10-CM: Other joint disorders (M20–M25)

ICD-9-CM: 736.7   Other acquired deformities of ankle and foot
ICD-10-CM: M21.6   Other acquired deformities of foot

ICD-9-CM: 729.2   Neuralgia, neuritis and radiculitis, unspecified
ICD-10-CM: M79.2   Neuralgia and neuritis, unspecified

Additions, Deletions, and Combinations

When chapter 13 of ICD-10-CM is compared with chapter 13 of ICD-9-CM, it is evident that many codes have been added, deleted, combined, or moved to another section or chapter. The following codes have been moved from a chapter in ICD-9-CM to chapter 13 of ICD-10-CM:

- Code 136.1, Behçet's syndrome, in ICD-9-CM chapter 1, Infectious and Parasitic Diseases, is classified to code M35.2, Behçet's disease, in ICD-10-CM chapter 13.

- Category code 274, Gout, in ICD-9-CM chapter 13, Endocrine, Nutritional and Metabolic Diseases and Immunity Disorders, is classified as a separate section, M10, Gout, in ICD-10-CM chapter 13.

- Code 268.2, Osteomalacia, in ICD-9-CM chapter 13 is classified to category code M83, Adult osteomalacia, in ICD-10-CM chapter 13.

- Code 446.0, Polyarteritis nodosa, in ICD-9-CM chapter 7, Diseases of the Circulatory System, is classified to category code M30, Polyarteritis nodosa and related conditions, in ICD-10-CM chapter 13.

- Code 446.21, Goodpasture's syndrome, in ICD-9-CM chapter 7, Diseases of the Circulatory System, is classified to code M31.0, Hypersensitivity angiitis, in ICD-10-CM chapter 13.

- Code 524.4, Malocclusion, unspecified, in ICD-9-CM chapter 9, Diseases of the Digestive System, is classified to code M26.4, Malocclusion, unspecified, in ICD-10-CM chapter 13.

- Code 836.x, Dislocation of patella, in ICD-9-CM chapter 17, Injury and Poisoning, is classified to category code M22, Disorder of patella, in ICD-10-CM chapter 13.

Following are some new categories and subcategories that are listed in chapter 13 of ICD-10-CM:

- M11.0, Hydroxyapatite deposition disease, has been expanded to include fifth- and sixth-character codes.

- M83, Adult osteomalacia, has additional fourth-character codes that specify manifestations of osteomalacia.

- M84.5, Pathologic fracture of bone in neoplastic disease, has been expanded to include specific sites as well as laterality.

- M85.1, Skeletal fluorosis, also specifies specific site and laterality.

- M86.2, Subacute osteomyelitis, is a separate section with fourth characters showing specific sites and fifth characters specifying laterality.

A new section in chapter 13, Intraoperative and postprocedural complications and disorders of the musculoskeletal system, not elsewhere classified (M96), is further divided into fourth, fifth, and even sixth characters. The fourth characters describe complications following surgery and postprocedural conditions (pseudoarthrosis after fusion or arthrodesis, postlaminectomy syndrome, postradiation kyphosis, postsurgical lordosis, and so on). The fifth characters further delineate the condition or complication (fracture of femur following insertion of orthopedic implant, joint prosthesis, or bone plate), and the sixth characters identify laterality, hemorrhage, hematoma, accidental puncture, and so on of these listed conditions.

Expansions

A number of codes for diseases of the musculoskeletal system and connective tissue have been expanded in ICD-10-CM. For example, rheumatoid arthritis and other inflammatory poly-arthropathies are classified to category code 714 in ICD-9-CM, but ICD-10-CM lists the following category codes to better reflect the specific types of arthritis:

M05 Rheumatoid arthritis with rheumatoid factor
M06 Other rheumatoid arthritis
M07 Enteropathic arthropathies
M08 Juvenile arthritis

Category M08 is further specified by four-, five-, and six-character codes indicating manifestations, specific sites, and laterality, respectively. Category M06 is further specified by four-, five-, and six-character codes indicating manifestations, specific sites, and laterality, respectively. Beginning with code M07.6, category M07 is further specified by fifth and sixth characters indicating specific sites and laterality, respectively. A note under M08 directs the user to code also any associated underlying condition, such as regional enteritis [Crohn's disease] (K50.–) and ulcerative colitis (K51.–). At the fourth-digit level in ICD-9-CM, unspecified juvenile rheumatoid arthritis is coded to 714.3 with fifth digits indicating chronic or unspecified, acute, and pauciarticular or monoarticular. In ICD-10-CM, this condition is further divided into fifth characters indicating specific sites and sixth characters specifying laterality.

Subcategory Codes Changed to Category Codes

Numerous subcategory codes in ICD-9-CM have been given a specific category code in ICD-10-CM and expanded at the fourth-, fifth-, or sixth-character level. For example:

ICD-9-CM: 710.0 Systemic lupus erythematosus
ICD-10-CM: M32   Systemic lupus erythematosus (SLE)
            M32.0 Drug-induced systemic lupus erythematosus
            M32.1 Systemic lupus erythematosus with organ or system involvement
                   M32.10 Systemic lupus erythematosus, organ or system involvement unspecified
                   M32.11 Endocarditis in systemic lupus erythematosus
                   M32.12 Pericarditis in systemic lupus erythematosus

	M32.13	Lung involvement in systemic lupus erythematosus
	M32.14	Glomerular disease in systemic lupus erythematosus
	M32.15	Tubulo-interstitial nephropathy in systemic lupus erythematosus
	M32.19	Other organ or system involvement in systemic lupus erythematosus

M32.8   Other forms of systemic lupus erythematosus

M32.9   Systemic lupus erythematosus, unspecified

ICD-9-CM: 710.3   Dermatomyositis
ICD-10-CM: M33   Dermatopolymyositis

M33.0   Juvenile dermatopolymyositis

M33.00   Juvenile dermatopolymyositis, organ involvement unspecified

M33.01   Juvenile dermatopolymyositis with respiratory involvement

M33.02   Juvenile dermatopolymyositis with myopathy

M33.09   Juvenile dermatopolymyositis with other organ involvement

M33.1   Other dermatopolymyositis

M33.10   Other dermatopolymyositis, organ involvement unspecified

M33.11   Other dermatopolymyositis with respiratory involvement

M33.12   Other dermatopolymyositis with myopathy

M33.19   Other dermatopolymyositis with other organ involvement

M33.2   Polymyositis

M33.20   Polymyositis, organ involvement unspecified

M33.21   Polymyositis with respiratory involvement

M33.22   Polymyositis with myopathy

M33.29   Polymyositis with other organ involvement

M33.9   Dermatopolymyositis, unspecified

M33.90   Dermatopolymyositis, unspecified, organ involvement unspecified

M33.91   Dermatopolymyositis, unspecified with respiratory involvement

M33.92   Dermatopolymyositis, unspecified with myopathy

M33.99   Dermatopolymyositis, unspecified with other organ involvement

CD-9-CM: 737.3   Kyphoscoliosis and scoliosis
ICD-10-CM: M41   Scoliosis

M41.0   Infantile idiopathic scoliosis

Note: Infantile is defined as birth through 4 years of age

M41.00   Infantile idiopathic scoliosis, site unspecified

M41.01   Infantile idiopathic scoliosis, occipito-atlanto-axial region

M41.02   Infantile idiopathic scoliosis, cervical region

M41.03   Infantile idiopathic scoliosis, cervicothoracic region

M41.04   Infantile idiopathic scoliosis, thoracic region

M41.05   Infantile idiopathic scoliosis, thoracolumbar region

M41.06　Infantile idiopathic scoliosis, lumbar region

M41.07　Infantile idiopathic scoliosis, lumbosacral region

M41.08　Infantile idiopathic scoliosis, sacral and sacrococcygeal region

M41.1　Juvenile and adolescent idiopathic scoliosis

M41.11　Juvenile idiopathic scoliosis

M41.111　Juvenile idiopathic scoliosis, occipito-atlanto-axial region

M41.112　Infantile idiopathic scoliosis, cervical region

M41.113　Infantile idiopathic scoliosis, cervicothoracic region

M41.114　Infantile idiopathic scoliosis, thoracic region

M41.115　Infantile idiopathic scoliosis, thoracolumbar region

M41.116　Infantile idiopathic scoliosis, lumbar region

M41.117　Infantile idiopathic scoliosis, lumbosacral region

M41.118　Infantile idiopathic scoliosis, sacral and sacrococcygeal region

M41.119　Infantile idiopathic scoliosis, site unspecified

Changes in these categories should be conveyed to physicians to make them aware of the documentation needed for accurate coding.

Expansion to Include Specific Sites and Laterality

Almost every code in chapter 13 of ICD-10-CM has been greatly expanded in some way. In many cases, the expansion includes very specific sites as well as laterality. For example:

ICD-9-CM:　729.5　Pain in limb

ICD-10-CM:　M79.6　Pain in limb, hand, foot, fingers and toes

M79.60　Pain in limb, unspecified

M79.601　Pain in right arm

M79.602　Pain in left arm

M79.603　Pain in arm, unspecified

M79.604　Pain in right leg

M79.605　Pain in left leg

M79.606　Pain in leg, unspecified

M79.609　Pain in unspecified limb

M79.62　Pain in upper arm

M79.621　Pain in right upper arm

M79.622　Pain in left upper arm

M79.629　Pain in unspecified upper arm

M79.63　Pain in forearm

M79.631　Pain in right forearm

M79.632　Pain in left forearm

M79.639　Pain in unspecified forearm

	M79.64	Pain in hand and fingers
		M79.641	Pain in right hand
		M79.642	Pain in left hand
		M79.643	Pain in unspecified hand
		M79.644	Pain in right finger(s)
		M79.645	Pain in left finger(s)
		M79.646	Pain in unspecified finger(s)

      M79.64   Pain in hand and fingers
            M79.641   Pain in right hand
            M79.642   Pain in left hand
            M79.643   Pain in unspecified hand
            M79.644   Pain in right finger(s)
            M79.645   Pain in left finger(s)
            M79.646   Pain in unspecified finger(s)

      M79.65   Pain in thigh
            M79.651   Pain in right thigh
            M79.652   Pain in left thigh
            M79.659   Pain in unspecified thigh

      M79.66   Pain in lower leg
            M79.661   Pain in right lower leg
            M79.662   Pain in left lower leg
            M79.669   Pain in unspecified lower leg

      M79.67   Pain in foot and toes
            M79.671   Pain in right foot
            M79.672   Pain in left foot
            M79.673   Pain in unspecified foot
            M79.674   Pain in right toe(s)
            M79.675   Pain in left toe(s)
            M79.676   Pain in unspecified toe(s)

   M79.8   Other specified soft tissue disorders
   M79.9   Soft tissue disorder, unspecified

Osteoporosis with Pathological Fracture

ICD-9-CM has no single code for osteoporosis with pathological fracture, but codes have been added in ICD-10-CM to classify these two conditions and to further identify additional types and sites of osteoporosis. Five- and six-character codes under these subcategories further delineate specific sites, and sixth characters specify laterality. For example:

ICD-9-CM: 733.0   Osteoporosis
ICD-10-CM: M80   Osteoporosis with current pathological fracture
                M80.0   Postmenopausal osteoporosis with current pathological fracture
                M80.8   Other osteoporosis with current pathological fracture
           M81   Osteoporosis without current pathological fracture
                M81.0   Postmenopausal osteoporosis without current pathological fracture
                M81.6   Localized osteoporosis [Lequesne]
                M81.8   Other osteoporosis without current pathological fracture

Extensions Added to Codes

Some category and subcategory codes in chapter 13 specify extensions that are to be added to each code. These extensions are listed as follows:

a   initial encounter for fracture
d   subsequent encounter for fracture with routine healing
g   subsequent encounter for fracture with delayed healing
j   subsequent encounter for fracture with nonunion

m   subsequent encounter for fracture with malunion

q   sequela

The category and subcategory codes that use these extensions are as follows:

M80   Osteoporosis with current pathological fracture

M84.3   Stress fracture

M84.4   Pathological fracture, not elsewhere classified

M84.5   Pathologic fracture of bone in neoplastic disease

M84.6   Pathologic fracture in other disease

Expansions to Include Notes

Some of the codes in chapter 13 of ICD-10-CM include notes indicating that an additional code should be assigned. For example:

M01   Direct infections of joint in infectious and parasitic diseases classified elsewhere
        Code first underlying disease, such as:
            leprosy [Hansen's disease] (A30.–)
            mycoses (B35–B49)
            O'nyong-nyong fever (A92.1)
            parathyroid fever (A01.1–A01.4)

M07   Enteropathic arthropathies
        Code also associated enteropathy, such as:
            regional enteritis [Crohn's disease] (K50.–)
            ulcerative colitis (K51.–)

M08   Juvenile arthritis
        Code also any associated underlying condition, such as:
            regional enteritis [Crohn's disease] (K50.–)
            ulcerative colitis (K51.–)

M36.0   Dermato(poly)myositis in neoplastic disease
        Code first underlying neoplasm (C00–D48)

M60.0   Infective myositis
        Use additional code (B95–B97) to identify infectious agent

M71.1   Other infective bursitis
        Use additional code (B95.–, B96.–) to identify causative organism

M65.0   Abscess of tendon sheath
        Use additional code (B95–B96) to identify bacterial agent

M87.1   Osteonecrosis due to drugs
        Code first (T36–T50) to identify drug

M94.3   Chondrolysis
        Code first any associated slipped upper femoral epiphysis (nontraumatic) (M93.0–)

Osteoarthritis

ICD-9-CM category 715 in ICD-9-CM, Osteoarthrosis and allied disorders, has fourth digits that specify whether the osteoarthrosis is primary, secondary, localized, and so on, and fifth digits indicate specific sites of the condition. In ICD-10-CM section M15 through M19, the classification for osteoarthritis is further divided into categories that specify types of osteoarthritis (polyosteoarthritis, osteoarthritis of hip, osteoarthritis of knee, osteoarthritis of first carpometacarpal joint, and other and unspecified osteoarthritis) at the fourth-character level and laterality at the fifth-character level.

Chapter 14

Diseases of the Genitourinary System

Chapter 14 of the ICD-10-CM Tabular List classifies diseases of the genitourinary system. It includes categories N00 through N99, which are arranged in the following blocks:

N00–N08   Glomerular diseases
N10–N16   Renal tubulo-interstitial diseases
N17–N19   Renal failure
N20–N23   Urolithiasis
N25–N29   Other disorders of kidney and ureter
N30–N39   Other diseases of the urinary system
N40–N51   Diseases of male genital organs
N60–N64   Disorders of breast
N70–N77   Inflammatory diseases of female pelvic organs
N80–N98   Noninflammatory disorders of female genital tract
N99   Other disorders of the genitourinary system

Title Changes

A number of block and category title changes have been made in chapter 14 of ICD-10-CM. A few examples of these changes include the following:

ICD-9-CM: 597   Urethritis, not sexually transmitted, and urethral syndrome
ICD-10-CM: N34   Urethritis and urethral syndrome

ICD-9-CM: 603   Hydrocele
ICD-10-CM: N43   Hydrocele and spermatocele

ICD-9-CM: Other Disorders of Female Genital Tract (617–629)
ICD-10-CM: Noninflammatory disorders of female genital tract (N80–N98)

ICD-9-CM: Nephritis, Nephrotic Syndrome, and Nephrosis (580–589)
ICD-10-CM: Glomerular diseases (N00–N08)

Additions, Deletions, and Combinations

When chapter 14 of ICD-10-CM is compared with chapter 10 in ICD-9-CM, it is evident that many codes have been added, deleted, combined, or moved to another section or chapter. Examples of codes moved from a chapter in ICD-9-CM to chapter 14 of ICD-10-CM include the following:

- Code 788.32, Stress incontinence (male), in ICD-9-CM chapter 16 is coded to N39.3, Stress incontinence (female) (male), in ICD-10-CM.

- Code 099.40, Nonspecific urethritis, in ICD-9-CM chapter 1, Infectious and Parasitic Diseases, is coded to N34.1, Nonspecific urethritis, in ICD-10-CM.

- Code 256.1, Hyperstimulation of ovaries, in ICD-9-CM chapter 3, Endocrine, Nutritional and Metabolic Diseases and Immunity Disorders, is coded to N98.1, Hyperstimulation of ovaries, in ICD-10-CM.

- Code 759.89, Hereditary nephropathy (759.89), in ICD-9-CM chapter 14, Congenital Anomalies, is coded to N07, Hereditary nephropathy, not elsewhere classified, in ICD-10-CM.

An example of a condition that no longer has its own code in ICD-10-CM is galactocele (ICD-9-CM code 611.5). In ICD-10-CM, this condition is simply coded to N64.8, Other specified disorders of the breast.

Code descriptions have been added in ICD-10-CM for vesicoureteral-reflux, with and without hydroureter.

ICD-9-CM:	593.7	Vesicoureteral reflux		
	593.70	Unspecified or without reflux nephropathy		
	593.71	With reflux nephropathy, unilateral		
	593.72	With reflux nephropathy, bilateral		
	593.73	With reflux nephropathy, not otherwise specified		
ICD-10-CM:	N13.7	Vesicoureteral-reflux		
	N13.70	Vesicoureteral-reflux, unspecified		
	N13.71	Vesicoureteral-reflux without reflux nephropathy		
	N13.72	Vesicoureteral-reflux with reflux nephropathy without hydroureter		
		N13.721	Vesicoureteral-reflux with reflux nephropathy without hydroureter, unilateral	
		N13.722	Vesicoureteral-reflux with reflux nephropathy without hydroureter, bilateral	
		N13.729	Vesicoureteral-reflux with reflux nephropathy without hydroureter, unspecified	
	N13.73	Vesicoureteral-reflux with reflux nephropathy with hydroureter		
		N13.731	Vesicoureteral-reflux with reflux nephropathy with hydroureter, unilateral	
		N13.732	Vesicoureteral-reflux with reflux nephropathy with hydroureter, bilateral	
		N13.739	Vesicoureteral-reflux with reflux nephropathy with hydroureter, unspecified	
	N13.8	Other obstructive and reflux uropathy		
	N13.9	Obstructive and reflux uropathy, unspecified		

ICD-10-CM has been restructured to bring together groups of conditions that are related by cause. For example, a new block for urolithiasis (N20–N23) further divides into separate categories for the specific calculus sites. In ICD-9-CM, there is no separate subchapter for urolithiasis, and the calculus sites are not grouped together.

> ICD-9-CM: Other Diseases of Urinary System (590–599)
> 592   Calculus of kidney and ureter
> 593   Other disorders of kidney and ureter
> 594   Calculus of lower urinary tract
> ICD-10-CM: Urolithiasis (N20–N23)
> N20   Calculus of kidney and ureter
> N21   Calculus of lower urinary tract
> N22   Calculus of urinary tract in diseases classified elsewhere

Finally, a new section in chapter 14, Intraoperative complications and postprocedural disorders of genitourinary system, not elsewhere classified (N99), is further divided into fourth, fifth, and even sixth characters. The fourth characters describe complications following surgery and postprocedural conditions (renal failure, urethral stricture, and so on). The fifth characters further delineate the condition or complication (complication of cystostomy, external stoma of urinary tract, and so on). The sixth characters identify hemorrhage, infection, malfunction, and so on.

Expansions

A number of codes for diseases of the genitourinary system have been expanded in ICD-10-CM.

Nodular Prostate

Code N40.1, Nodular prostate, includes fifth characters to indicate whether obstruction, hematuria, or some other complication is present. For example:

> ICD-9-CM: 600.1   Nodular prostate
> ICD-10-CM: N40.1   Nodular prostate
> N40.10   Nodular prostate without complication
> N40.11   Nodular prostate with obstruction
> N40.12   Nodular prostate with hematuria
> N40.13   Nodular prostate with obstruction and hematuria
> N40.19   Nodular prostate with other complication

Subcategory Codes Changed to Category Codes

Numerous codes included as subcategory codes in ICD-9-CM have been given specific category codes in ICD-10-CM and expanded at the fourth- or fifth-character level. For example:

> ICD-9-CM: 599.7   Hematura
> ICD-10-CM: N02   Recurrent and persistent hematuria
> N02.0   Recurrent and persistent hematuria with minor glomerular abnormality
> N02.1   Recurrent and persistent hematuria with focal and segmental glomerular lesions
> N02.2   Recurrent and persistent hematuria with diffuse membranous glomerulonephritis

> N02.3 Recurrent and persistent hematuria with diffuse mesangial proliferative glomerulonephritis
> N02.4 Recurrent and persistent hematuria with diffuse endocapillary proliferative glomerulonephritis
> N02.5 Recurrent and persistent hematuria with diffuse esangiocapillary glomerulonephritis
> N02.6 Recurrent and persistent hematuria with dense deposit disease
> N02.7 Recurrent and persistent hematuria with diffuse crescentic glomerulonephritis
> N02.8 Recurrent and persistent hematuria with other morphologic changes
> N02.9 Recurrent and persistent hematuria with unspecified morphologic changes

ICD-9-CM:	622.1	Dysplasia of cervix (uteri)
ICD-10-CM:	N87	Dysplasia of cervix uteri
	N87.0	Mild cervical dysplasia
	N87.1	Moderate cervical dysplasia
	N87.2	Severe cervical dysplasia, not elsewhere classified
	N87.9	Dysplasia of cervix uteri, unspecified

ICD-9-CM:	614.0	Acute salpingitis and oophoritis
	614.1	Chronic salpingitis and oophoritis
	614.2	Salpingitis and oophoritis not specified as acute, subacute, or chronic
ICD-10-CM:	N70	Salpingitis and oophoritis
	N70.0	Acute salpingitis and oophoritis
	N70.01	Acute salpingitis
	N70.02	Acute oophoritis
	N70.03	Acute salpingitis and oophoritis
	N70.1	Chronic salpingitis and oophoritis
	N70.11	Chronic salpingitis
	N70.12	Chronic oophoritis
	N70.13	Chronic salpingitis and oophoritis
	N70.9	Salpingitis and oophoritis, unspecified
	N70.91	Salpingitis, unspecified
	N70.92	Oophoritis, unspecified
	N70.93	Salpingitis and oophoritis, unspecified

Changes in these categories should be conveyed to physicians to make them aware of the documentation needed for accurate coding.

Chronic Renal Failure

In ICD-9-CM, code 585, Chronic renal failure, stands as a category code only. In contrast, ICD-10-CM, category N18, Chronic renal failure, is further divided into fourth characters indicating the following:

> N18 Chronic renal failure
> N18.0 End-stage renal disease
> N18.8 Other chronic renal failure
> N18.9 Chronic renal failure, unspecified

Benign Mammary Dysplasia

Category N60, Benign mammary dysplasia, has been expanded in ICD-10-CM to include fifth characters to indicate male or female breast conditions as well as laterality. For example:

ICD-9-CM: 610.3   Fibrosclerosis of breast
ICD-10-CM: N60.3   Fibrosclerosis of breast
               N60.30   Fibrosclerosis of female breast, unspecified side
               N60.31   Fibrosclerosis of right female breast
               N60.32   Fibrosclerosis of left female breast
               N60.33   Fibrosclerosis of right male breast
               N60.34   Fibrosclerosis of left male breast
               N60.35   Fibrosclerosis of male breast, unspecified side

Other Noninflammatory Disorders of Vagina

In ICD-10-CM, category N89, Other noninflammatory disorders of vagina, is further divided at the fourth-character level to specify stages of dysplasia. In ICD-9-CM, subcategory code 623.0, Dysplasia of vagina, does not specify the stages. For example:

ICD-9-CM: 623.0   Dysplasia of vagina
ICD-10-CM: N89   Other noninflammatory disorders of vagina
               N89.0   Mild vaginal dysplasia
               N89.1   Moderate vaginal dysplasia
               N89.2   Severe vaginal dysplasia, not elsewhere classified
               N89.3   Dysplasia of vagina, unspecified

Expansion to Include Notes

Some of the categories in chapter 14 of ICD-10-CM have been expanded to include notes indicating that an additional code should be used. For example:

N11   Chronic tubulo-interstitial nephritis
        Use additional code (B95–B97) to identify infectious agent

N14   Drug- and heavy-metal-induced tubulo-interstitial and tubular conditions
        Code first (T36–T65) to identify drug and toxic agent

N17   Acute renal failure
        Code also associated underlying condition

N18   Chronic renal failure
        Code also associated underlying condition

Chapter 15

Conditions Related to Pregnancy and Childbirth

Chapter 15 of the ICD-10-CM Tabular List provides codes for pregnancy, childbirth, and conditions arising during the puerperium. It includes categories O00 through O99, which are arranged in the following blocks:

O00–O08	Pregnancy with abortive outcome
O09	Supervision of high-risk pregnancy
O10–O16	Edema, proteinuria and hypertensive disorders in pregnancy, childbirth and the puerperium
O20–O29	Other maternal disorders predominantly related to pregnancy
O30–O48	Maternal care related to the fetus and amniotic cavity and possible delivery problems
O60–O77	Complications of labor and delivery
O80, O82	Encounter for delivery
O85–O92	Complications predominantly related to the puerperium
O93	Sequelae of complication of pregnancy, childbirth, and the puerperium
O94–O99	Other obstetric conditions, not elsewhere classified

Codes from chapter 15 of ICD-10-CM are to be used with the records of mothers and never with the records of newborns. Codes from category O37, Fetal care for fetal abnormality and damage, may be used either on a mother's record or on a record created for a fetus, depending on the record-keeping system of the facility.

In a significant departure from ICD-9-CM, in ICD-10-CM fifth- and sixth-character subclassifications identify the trimester in which the condition occurs. Trimesters are counted from the first day of the last menstrual period and are defined as follows:

- First trimester: less than 14 weeks 0 days of gestation

- Second trimester: 14 weeks 0 days to less than 28 weeks 0 days of gestation

- Third trimester: 28 weeks 0 days gestation until delivery

Title Changes

A number of category title changes have been made in chapter 15. A few examples of these changes include the following:

| ICD-9-CM: | 654 | Abnormality of organs and soft tissues of pelvis |
| ICD-10-CM: | O34 | Maternal care for abnormality of pelvic organs |

| ICD-9-CM: | 644 | Early or threatened labor |
| ICD-10-CM: | O47 | False labor |

| ICD-9-CM: | 664 | Trauma to perineum and vulva during delivery |
| ICD-10-CM: | O70 | Perineal laceration during delivery |

Additions, Deletions, and Combinations

When chapter 15 of ICD-10-CM is compared with chapter 11 of ICD-9-CM, it is evident that many codes have been added, deleted, combined, or moved to another section or chapter. For example:

Pregnancy with abortive outcome (O00–O08)
O00 Ectopic pregnancy
O01 Hydatidiform mole
O02 Other abnormal products of conception
O03 Spontaneous abortion
O04 Complications following (induced) termination of pregnancy
O07 Failed attempted termination of pregnancy
O08 Complications following ectopic and molar pregnancy

Fourth characters under O03, Spontaneous abortion, indicate whether the abortion was complete or incomplete and whether it was complicated. ICD-10-CM provides fewer complication codes than ICD-9-CM does. Some examples of these codes from O03 include:

O03.0 Incomplete spontaneous abortion complicated by genitourinary tract and pelvic infection
O03.1 Incomplete spontaneous abortion complicated by delayed or excessive hemorrhage
O03.2 Incomplete spontaneous abortion complicated by embolism
O03.3 Incomplete spontaneous abortion with other and unspecified complications
O03.4 Incomplete spontaneous abortion without complication
O03.5 Complete or unspecified spontaneous abortion complicated by genitourinary tract and pelvic infection
O03.6 Complete or unspecified spontaneous abortion complicated by delayed or excessive hemorrhage
O03.7 Complete or unspecified spontaneous abortion complicated by embolism
O03.8 Complete or unspecified spontaneous abortion with other and unspecified complications
O03.9 Complete or unspecified spontaneous abortion without complication

Codes for elective (legal or therapeutic) abortion are classified with the abortion codes in ICD-9-CM. The abortion codes have been moved to code Z33.2, Encounter for elective termination of pregnancy, in chapter 21 of ICD-10-CM.

Category O04, Complications following (induced) termination of pregnancy, is used when there are complications of termination of pregnancy. Fourth characters indicate the complications. For example:

O04   Complications following (induced) termination of pregnancy
    Includes: complications following (induced) termination of pregnancy
    Excludes 1:   encounter for elective termination of pregnancy, uncomplicated (Z33.2)
                failed attempted termination of pregnancy (O07.–)
    O04.5   Termination of pregnancy complicated by genitourinary tract and pelvic infection
    O04.6   Termination of pregnancy complicated by delayed or excessive hemorrhage
    O04.7   Termination of pregnancy complicated by embolism
    O04.8   Termination of pregnancy with other and unspecified complications
            O04.80   Termination of pregnancy with unspecified complications
            O04.89   Termination of pregnancy with other complications

Category O08, Complications following ectopic and molar pregnancy, is used with categories O00 through O02 to identify associated complications. For example:

O08.0   Genitourinary tract and pelvic infection following ectopic and molar pregnancy
O08.1   Delayed or excessive hemorrhage following ectopic and molar pregnancy
O08.2   Embolism following ectopic and molar pregnancy
O08.3   Shock following ectopic and molar pregnancy
O08.4   Renal failure following ectopic and molar pregnancy
O08.5   Metabolic disorders following an ectopic and molar pregnancy
O08.6   Damage to pelvic organs and tissues following ectopic and molar pregnancy
O08.7   Other venous complications following ectopic and molar pregnancy
O08.8   Other complications following ectopic and molar pregnancy
        O08.81   Cardiac arrest following ectopic and molar pregnancy
        O08.82   Sepsis following ectopic and molar pregnancy
        O08.83   Urinary tract infection following an ectopic and molar pregnancy
        O08.89   Other complications following ectopic and molar pregnancy
O08.9   Unspecified complication following ectopic and molar pregnancy

Code selection for supervision of high-risk pregnancy requires documentation of the trimester in which the treatment occurred. For example:

O09   Supervision of high-risk pregnancy
    O09.0   Supervision of pregnancy with history of infertility
        O09.00   Supervision of pregnancy with history of infertility, unspecified
                trimester
        O09.01   Supervision of pregnancy with history of infertility, first trimester
        O09.02   Supervision of pregnancy with history of infertility, second trimester
        O09.03   Supervision with history of infertility, third trimester

The other fourth-character subcategory codes in this category include:

O09.1   Supervision of pregnancy with history of ectopic or molar pregnancy
O09.2   Supervision of pregnancy with other poor reproductive or obstetric history
O09.3   Supervision of pregnancy with insufficient antenatal care
O09.4   Supervision of pregnancy with grand multiparity
O09.5   Supervision of elderly primigravida and multigravida
        Pregnancy for a female 35 years and older at expected date of delivery
O09.6   Supervision of young primigravida and multigravida
        Supervision of pregnancy for a female less than 16 years old at expected date of delivery
O09.7   Supervision of high-risk pregnancy due to social problems
O09.8   Supervision of other high-risk pregnancies
O09.9   Supervision of high-risk pregnancy, unspecified

Within this category, new areas of high-risk have been assigned codes. Fifth and sixth characters in each of these subcategories reflect the trimester in which treatment is sought. In ICD-9-CM, the V code for high-risk pregnancy is located in the Supplementary Classification.

Expansions

A number of codes for pregnancy, childbirth, and conditions arising during the puerperium have been expanded in ICD-10-CM.

Hypertension Complicating Pregnancy, Childbirth, and the Puerperium

ICD-9-CM category code 642, Hypertension complicating pregnancy, childbirth and the puerperium, has been expanded in ICD-10-CM. In fact, a block of category codes—Edema, proteinuria and hypertensive disorders in pregnancy, childbirth and the puerperium (O10–O16)—has been created to cover these conditions.

O10   Pre-existing hypertension complicating pregnancy, childbirth and the puerperium
O11   Pre-existing hypertensive disorder with superimposed proteinuria
O12   Gestational [pregnancy-induced] edema and proteinuria without hypertension
O13   Gestational [pregnancy-induced] hypertension without significant proteinuria
O14   Gestational [pregnancy-induced] hypertension with significant proteinuria
O15   Eclampsia
O16   Unspecified maternal hypertension

Within category code O10, fourth characters indicate the exact nature of the hypertension; fifth characters indicate whether the hypertension complicates the pregnancy, the childbirth, or the puerperium; and sixth characters indicate the trimester involved. For example:

O10.1   Pre-existing hypertensive heart disease complicating pregnancy, childbirth and the puerperium
    O10.11   Pre-existing hypertensive heart disease complicating pregnancy
        O10.111   Pre-existing hypertensive heart disease complicating pregnancy, first trimester
        O10.112   Pre-existing hypertensive heart disease complicating pregnancy, second trimester
        O10.113   Pre-existing hypertensive heart disease complicating pregnancy, third trimester
        O10.119   Pre-existing hypertensive heart disease complicating pregnancy, trimester unspecified
    O10.12   Pre-existing hypertensive heart disease complicating childbirth
    O10.13   Pre-existing hypertensive heart disease complicating the puerperium

The presence or absence of proteinuria is important for the physician to document in order to accurately assign the ICD-10-CM code.

Unspecified maternal hypertension, including transient hypertension of pregnancy, is reported to category O16, Unspecified maternal hypertension.

Hyperemesis Gravidarum

Another significant change in ICD-10-CM is that the time period specified for differentiating between early vomiting and late vomiting is 20 completed weeks rather than 22 completed weeks as in ICD-9-CM:

> O21 Excessive vomiting in pregnancy
> > O21.0 Mild hyperemesis gravidarum
> > Hyperemesis gravidarum, mild or unspecified, starting before the end of the 20th week of gestation
> > O21.2 Late vomiting of pregnancy
> > Excessive vomiting starting after 20 completed weeks of gestation

Expansions to Add Specifity

Many of the codes in ICD-10-CM are much more specific than the same codes in ICD-9-CM. A few examples include the following:

> ICD-9-CM: 646.6 Infections of genitourinary tract in pregnancy
> ICD-10-CM: O23 Infections of genitourinary tract in pregnancy
> Use additional code to identify organism (B95.–, B96.–)
> > O23.0 Infections of kidney in pregnancy
> > > O23.00 Infections of kidney in pregnancy, unspecified trimester
> > > O23.01 Infections of kidney in pregnancy, first trimester
> > > O23.02 Infections of kidney in pregnancy, second trimester
> > > O23.03 Infections of kidney in pregnancy, third trimester
> > O23.1 Infections of bladder in pregnancy
> > > O23.10 Infections of bladder in pregnancy, unspecified trimester
> > > O23.11 Infections of bladder in pregnancy, first trimester
> > > O23.12 Infections of bladder in pregnancy, second trimester
> > > O23.13 Infections of bladder in pregnancy, third trimester
> > O23.2 Infections of urethra in pregnancy
> > > O23.20 Infections of urethra in pregnancy, unspecified trimester
> > > O23.21 Infections of urethra in pregnancy, first trimester
> > > O23.22 Infections of urethra in pregnancy, second trimester
> > > O23.23 Infections of urethra in pregnancy, third trimester

Additional fourth-character subcategories identify other genitourinary sites. Fifth characters identify the trimester in which the patient is seeking treatment. For example:

> ICD-9-CM: 641.2 Premature separation of placenta
> ICD-10-CM: O45 Premature separation of placenta [abruptio placentae]
> > O45.0 Premature separation of placenta with coagulation defect
> > > O45.00 Premature separation of placenta with coagulation defect, unspecified
> > > > O45.001 Premature separation of placenta with coagulation defect, unspecified, first trimester
> > > > O45.002 Premature separation of placenta with coagulation defect, unspecified, second trimester

O45.003	Premature separation of placenta with coagulation defect, unspecified, third trimester
O45.009	Premature separation of placenta with coagulation defect, unspecified, unspecified trimester
O45.01	Premature separation of placenta with afibrinogenemia
O45.02	Premature separation of placenta with disseminated intravascular coagulation
O45.09	Premature separation of placenta with other coagulation defect

Sixth characters in O45.0 through O45.8 identify the trimester in which treatment is being sought. Fifth characters in O45.9 identify the trimester.

Diabetes Mellitus in Pregnancy, Childbirth, and the Puerperium

The codes for diabetes mellitus in pregnancy, childbirth, and the puerperium have been greatly expanded in ICD-10-CM. Fourth-character subcategory codes identify the type of diabetes as preexisting (type 1, type 2, or unspecified) or gestational. Fifth characters indicate whether the diabetes is treated during pregnancy, childbirth, or the puerperium. Sixth characters for pre-existing diabetes indicate the trimester during which treatment is sought. Sixth characters for gestational diabetes identify whether the gestational diabetes mellitus is diet controlled, insulin controlled, or unspecified control. Examples of some of the codes for diabetes include:

O24   Diabetes mellitus in pregnancy, childbirth and the puerperium
    O24.0   Pre-existing diabetes mellitus, type 1, in pregnancy, childbirth and the puerperium
        Juvenile onset diabetes mellitus, in pregnancy, childbirth and the puerperium
        Ketosis-prone diabetes mellitus in pregnancy, childbirth and the puerperium
        Use additional code from category E10 to further identify any manifestations
        O24.01   Pre-existing diabetes mellitus, type 1, in pregnancy
            O24.011   Pre-existing diabetes mellitus, type 1, in pregnancy, first trimester
            O24.012   Pre-existing diabetes mellitus, type 1, in pregnancy, second trimester
            O24.013   Pre-existing diabetes mellitus, type 1, in pregnancy, third trimester
            O24.019   Pre-existing diabetes mellitus, type 1, in pregnancy, unspecified trimester
        O24.02   Pre-existing diabetes mellitus, type 1, in childbirth
        O24.03   Pre-existing diabetes mellitus, type 1, in the puerperium

Users are reminded to identify any manifestations of the diabetes by notes that direct them to use additional codes.

Complications of Pregnancy, Not Elsewhere Classified

The number of codes used to describe other complications of pregnancy not elsewhere classified has been increased. Many conditions that are coded to ICD-9-CM code 646.8, Other specified complications of pregnancy, have been given distinct codes in ICD-10-CM. For example:

O26.0	Excessive weight gain in pregnancy
O26.1	Low weight gain in pregnancy
O26.2	Pregnancy care of habitual aborter
O26.3	Retained intrauterine contraceptive device in pregnancy
O26.4	Herpes gestationis
O26.5	Maternal hypotension syndrome
O26.6	Liver disorders in pregnancy, childbirth and the puerperium
O26.7	Subluxation of symphis (pubis) in pregnancy, childbirth and the puerperium
O26.8	Other specified pregnancy-related complications
O26.81	Pregnancy-related exhaustion and fatigue
O26.82	Pregnancy-related peripheral neuritis
O26.83	Pregnancy-related renal disease
O26.84	Uterine size–date discrepancy complicating pregnancy
O26.89	Other specified pregnancy-related conditions
O26.9	Pregnancy-related condition, unspecified

Fifth and sometimes sixth characters identify the trimester.

Other Maternal Diseases Classifiable Elsewhere But Complicating Pregnancy, Childbirth, and the Puerperium

Category O99, Other maternal diseases classifiable elsewhere but complicating pregnancy, childbirth and the puerperium, includes many of the conditions coded to ICD-9-CM categories 647 and 648, but with additional detail. The subcategory codes in O99 are:

O99.0	Anemia complicating pregnancy, childbirth and the puerperium
O99.1	Other diseases of blood and blood-forming organs and certain disorders involving the immune mechanism complicating pregnancy, childbirth and the puerperium
O99.2	Endocrine, nutritional and metabolic diseases complicating pregnancy, childbirth and the puerperium
O99.3	Mental disorders and diseases of the nervous system complicating pregnancy, childbirth and the puerperium
O99.4	Diseases of the circulatory system complicating pregnancy, childbirth and the puerperium
O99.5	Diseases of the respiratory system complicating pregnancy, childbirth and the puerperium
O99.6	Diseases of the digestive system complicating pregnancy, childbirth and the puerperium
O99.7	Diseases of the skin and subcutaneous tissue complicating pregnancy, childbirth and the puerperium
O99.8	Other specified diseases and conditions complicating pregnancy, childbirth and the puerperium

Many of these subcategory codes have fifth and sixth characters that provide specificity. In addition, users are instructed to assign an additional code to identify the specific condition. For example:

O99.3   Mental disorders and diseases of the nervous system complicating pregnancy, childbirth and the puerperium

O99.31   Alcohol use complicating pregnancy, childbirth and the puerperium
Use additional code(s) from F10 to identify manifestations of the alcohol use

O99.310   Alcohol use complicating pregnancy, first trimester
O99.311   Alcohol use complicating pregnancy, second trimester
O99.312   Alcohol use complicating pregnancy, third trimester
O99.313   Alcohol use complicating pregnancy, unspecified trimester
O99.314   Alcohol use complicating childbirth
O99.315   Alcohol use complicating the puerperium

O99.7   Diseases of the skin and subcutaneous tissue complicating pregnancy, childbirth and the puerperium

O99.71   Pruritic urticarial papules and plaques of pregnancy (PUPPP)

O99.711   Pruritic urticarial papules and plaques of pregnancy (PUPPP), first trimester
O99.712   Pruritic urticarial papules and plaques of pregnancy (PUPPP), second trimester
O99.713   Pruritic urticarial papules and plaques of pregnancy (PUPPP), third trimester
O99.719   Pruritic urticarial papules and plaques of pregnancy (PUPPP), unspecified trimester

Abnormal Findings on Antenatal Screening of Mother

Category O28, Abnormal findings on antenatal screening of mother, identifies various types of abnormal findings discovered through antenatal screening. For example:

O28.0   Abnormal hematological finding on antenatal screening of mother
O28.1   Abnormal biochemical finding on antenatal screening of mother
O28.2   Abnormal cytological finding on antenatal screening of mother
O28.3   Abnormal ultrasonic finding on antenatal screening of mother

Complications of Anesthesia

There are substantial changes in ICD-10-CM for coding complications of anesthesia. In ICD-9-CM, category 668, Complications of the administration of anesthetic or other sedation in labor and delivery, is used to classify these types of complications. In ICD-10-CM, three separate rubrics are used to classify anesthetic complications, depending on when the anesthesia is used.

Category O29 is used to code complications of anesthesia or other sedation during pregnancy. Examples of codes from category O29 include:

O29   Complications of anesthesia during pregnancy
Includes: maternal complications arising from the administration of a general, regional or local anesthetic, analgesic or other sedation during pregnancy
Use additional code, if necessary, to identify the complication
Excludes 2:   complications of anesthesia during labor and delivery (O74.–)
complications of anesthesia during the puerperium (O89.–)

O29.0   Pulmonary complications of anesthesia during pregnancy

O29.0x   Pulmonary complications of anesthesia during pregnancy

O29.0x1   Pulmonary complications of anesthesia during pregnancy, first trimester

O29.0x2 Pulmonary complications of anesthesia during pregnancy, second trimester

O29.0x3 Pulmonary complications of anesthesia during pregnancy, third trimester

O29.0x9 Pulmonary complications of anesthesia during pregnancy, unspecified trimester

Some of the other fourth-character subcategories include:

O29.1 Cardiac complications of anesthesia during pregnancy
O29.2 Central nervous system complications of anesthesia during pregnancy
O29.5 Other complications of spinal and epidural anesthesia during pregnancy
O29.8 Other complications of anesthesia during pregnancy
O29.9 Unspecified complications of anesthesia during pregnancy

There are three other new codes in category O29:

O29.3 Toxic reaction to local anesthesia during pregnancy
O29.4 Spinal and epidural anesthesia-induced headache during pregnancy
O29.6 Failed or difficult intubation for anesthesia during pregnancy

Each has fifth and possibly sixth characters to provide additional specificity.

Category O74, Complications of anesthesia during labor and delivery, is used to code complications of anesthesia or other sedation during labor and delivery. The coding professional is reminded to use an additional code to identify the specific complication. Finally, code O89 is used to code complications of anesthesia during the puerperium, and, again, users are reminded to use an additional code to identify the specific complication.

Multiple Gestations

As in ICD-9-CM, multiple gestations are coded in ICD-10-CM:

O30 Multiple gestation
   Use additional code(s) to identify any complications specific to multiple gestation
  O30.0 Twin pregnancy
  O30.1 Triplet pregnancy
  O30.2 Quadruplet pregnancy
  O30.8 Other multiple gestation

Fifth and sixth characters add increased specificity.

In addition, category O31 is used to identify complications specific to multiple gestation. For example:

O31 Complications specific to multiple gestation
  O31.0 Papyraceous fetus
  O31.1 Continuing pregnancy after spontaneous abortion of one fetus or more
  O31.2 Continuing pregnancy after intrauterine death of one fetus or more
  O31.3 Continuing pregnancy after other abortion of one fetus or more
  O31.8 Other complications specific to multiple gestation

Fifth and sixth characters add information about the trimester in which the complication occurs.

ICD-10-CM provides extensions that are used to identify the fetus to which a complication code applies. For example, extension 1 refers to fetus A, extension 2 to fetus B, and so on.

Fetal Care for Fetal Abnormality and Damage

Category O37, Fetal care for fetal abnormality and damage, is used with the mother's record or a record created for the fetus, depending on the record-keeping system of the facility where treatment is provided. The codes in this category would not be used on a newborn's record. Codes from category O37 include:

O37.0   Fetal care for fetal abnormality
O37.1   Complication to fetus from fetal care for fetal abnormality

Premature Rupture of Membranes

Category O42, Premature rupture of membranes, includes fourth characters to identify the length of time between the rupture and the onset of delivery and fifth characters to identify the weeks of gestation at the time the membranes ruptured. Sixth characters for rupture of membranes before 37 completed weeks of gestation identify the trimester in which rupture occurred. For example:

O42.0   Premature rupture of membranes, onset of labor within 24 hours of rupture
    O42.00   Premature rupture of membranes, onset of labor within 24 hours of rupture, unspecified weeks of gestation
    O42.01   Preterm premature rupture of membranes, onset of labor within 24 hours of rupture
    Premature rupture of membranes before 37 completed weeks of gestation
        O42.011   Preterm premature rupture of membranes, onset of labor within 24 hours of rupture, first trimester
        O42.012   Preterm premature rupture of membranes, onset of labor within 24 hours of rupture, second trimester
        O42.013   Preterm premature rupture of membranes, onset of labor within 24 hours of rupture, third trimester
        O42.019   Preterm premature rupture of membranes, onset of labor within 24 hours of rupture, unspecified trimester
    O42.02   Full-term premature rupture of membranes, onset of labor within 24 hours of rupture
    Premature rupture of membranes after 37 completed weeks of gestation

Antepartum Hemorrhage

The codes for antepartum hemorrhage have been expanded in ICD-10-CM. Code O46, Antepartum hemorrhage, not elsewhere classified, has fourth characters that indicate hemorrhage with coagulation defect and other antepartum hemorrhage. Specific types of coagulation defects are classified such as afibrinogenemia, disseminated intravascular coagulation, and other coagulation defect. For example:

O46.0   Antepartum hemorrhage with coagulation defect
    O46.00   Antepartum hemorrhage with coagulation defect, unspecified
        O46.001   Antepartum hemorrhage with coagulation defect, unspecified, first trimester

O46.002   Antepartum hemorrhage with coagulation defect, unspecified, second trimester

O46.003   Antepartum hemorrhage with coagulation defect, unspecified, third trimester

O46.009   Antepartum hemorrhage with coagulation defect, unspecified, unspecified trimester

O46.01   Antepartum hemorrhage with afibrinogenemia

O46.011   Antepartum hemorrhage with afibrinogenemia, first trimester

O46.012   Antepartum hemorrhage with afibrinogenemia, second trimester

O46.013   Antepartum hemorrhage with afibrinogenemia, third trimester

O46.019   Antepartum hemorrhage with afibrinogenemia, unspecified trimester

This information should be documented in the patient's health record.

Obstructed Labor

The ICD-10-CM codes for obstructed labor incorporate the reason for the obstruction into the code; thus, only one code is required rather than two as in ICD-9-CM. For example, to code obstructed labor due to breech presentation, the following ICD-9-CM codes are used: 660.0x, Obstruction caused by malposition of fetus at onset of labor, and 652.2x, Breech presentation without mention of version. In ICD-10-CM, only code O64.1, Obstructed labor due to breech presentation, is used.

Uncomplicated Delivery

Category O80 is used in ICD-10-CM to code an encounter for a full-term uncomplicated delivery. This code is for use as a single diagnosis code and is not to be used with any other code from chapter 15. Uncomplicated delivery is defined as one requiring minimal or no assistance, with or without episiotomy, without fetal manipulation or instrumentation (forceps) of a spontaneous, cephalic, vaginal, full-term, single, live-born infant. An outcome of delivery code from chapter 21 can be used with this code.

There is no specific code in ICD-9-CM for a malignant neoplasm complicating pregnancy, childbirth, or the puerperium, but ICD-10-CM provides a new subcategory to classify this type of condition under category code O94, Maternal malignant neoplasms, traumatic injuries and abuse classifiable elsewhere but complicating pregnancy, childbirth and the puerperium. An example of a new neoplasm code is O94.111, Malignant neoplasm complicating pregnancy, first trimester. Users are instructed to use an additional code to identify the neoplasm.

Also in this category are codes for injury, poisoning, and other consequences of external causes complicating pregnancy, childbirth, and the puerperium. Once again, users are instructed to use an additional code to identify the injury or poisoning. An example of a code in this subcategory is O94.211, Injury, poisoning and certain other consequences of external causes complicating pregnancy, first trimester.

Finally, there are codes to identify physical, sexual, or psychological abuse complicating pregnancy, childbirth, and the puerperium. An example is O94.511, Psychological abuse complicating pregnancy, first trimester.

Chapter 16

Conditions Originating in the Perinatal Period

Chapter 16 the ICD-10-CM Tabular List classifies certain conditions originating during the perinatal period. It includes categories P00 through P96, which are arranged in the following blocks:

P00–P04   Newborn affected by maternal factors and by complications of pregnancy, labor and delivery
P05–P08   Disorders of newborn related to length of gestation and fetal growth
P10–P15   Birth trauma
P19–P29   Respiratory and cardiovascular disorders specific to the perinatal period
P35–P39   Infections specific to the perinatal period
P50–P61   Hemorrhagic and hematological disorders of newborn
P70–P74   Transitory endocrine and metabolic disorders specific to newborn
P75–P78   Digestive system disorders of newborn
P80–P83   Conditions involving the integument and temperature regulation of newborn
P84   Other problems with newborn
P90–P96   Other disorders originating in the perinatal period

Codes from this chapter are for use with the records of newborns only and are never used with the records of mothers.

Title Changes

A number of block and category title changes have been made in chapter 16 of ICD-10-CM. A few examples of these changes include the following:

ICD-9-CM: Maternal Causes of Perinatal Morbidity and Mortality (760–763)
ICD-10-CM: Newborn affected by maternal factors and by complications of pregnancy, labor and delivery (P00–P04)

ICD-9-CM: 760   Fetus or newborn affected by maternal conditions which may be unrelated to present pregnancy
ICD-10-CM: P00   Newborn (suspected to be) affected by maternal conditions that may be unrelated to present pregnancy

The phrase *fetus or newborn* used in many ICD-9-CM codes is not used in ICD-10-CM. Also, in the first block in ICD-10-CM chapter 16, Newborn affected by maternal factors and by complications of pregnancy, labor and delivery (P00–P04), the word *suspected* is included in the code titles (as a nonessential modifier) to indicate that the codes are for use when the listed maternal conditions are specified as the cause of confirmed or suspected newborn morbidity or potential morbidity.

Additions, Deletions, and Combinations

Code P04, Newborn (suspected to be) affected by noxious influences transmitted via placenta or breast milk, includes codes for newborns affected by maternal anesthesia and analgesia, by maternal use of tobacco, by chemical substances, and by other maternal medications such as cancer chemotherapy. For example:

P04   Newborn (suspected to be) affected by noxious influences transmitted via placenta or breast milk
    P04.0   Newborn (suspected to be) affected by maternal anesthesia and analgesia in pregnancy, labor and delivery
    P04.1   Newborn (suspected to be) affected by other maternal medication
    P04.2   Newborn (suspected to be) affected by maternal use of tobacco
    P04.3   Newborn (suspected to be) affected by maternal use of alcohol
    P04.4   Newborn (suspected to be) affected by maternal use of drugs of addiction
       P04.41   Newborn (suspected to be) affected by maternal use of cocaine
       P04.49   Newborn (suspected to be) affected by maternal use of other drugs of addiction
    P04.5   Newborn (suspected to be) affected by maternal use of nutritional chemical substances
    P04.6   Newborn (suspected to be) affected by maternal exposure to environmental chemical substances
    P04.8   Newborn (suspected to be) affected by other maternal noxious substances
    P04.9   Newborn (suspected to be) affected by maternal noxious substance, unspecified

Slow Fetal Growth and Fetal Malnutrition

There have been changes in the codes to identify slow fetal growth and fetal malnutrition. Two separate codes identify light for gestational age and small for gestational age. Physicians will need to make a distinction between these two conditions in their documentation.

P05   Disorders of newborn related to slow fetal growth and fetal malnutrition
    P05.0   Newborn light for gestational age
           Newborn light-for-dates
       P05.00   Newborn light for gestational age, unspecified weight
       P05.01   Newborn light for gestational age, less than 500 grams
       P05.02   Newborn light for gestational age, 500–749 grams
    P05.1   Newborn small for gestational age
           Newborn small-and-light-for-dates
           Newborn small-for-dates
       P05.10   Newborn small for gestational age, unspecified weight
       P05.11   Newborn small for gestational age, less than 500 grams
       P05.12   Newborn small for gestational age, 500–749 grams
    P05.2   Newborn affected by fetal (intrauterine) malnutrition not light or small for gestational age
    P05.9   Newborn affected by slow intrauterine growth, unspecified

There are other fifth characters under P05.0 and P05.1 for weight up to 2499 grams.

Codes P07.0 and P07.1 identify low-birth-weight newborns when the low birth weight is not due to slow fetal growth or fetal malnutrition. For example:

P07 Disorders of newborn related to short gestation and low birth weight, not elsewhere classified

 Note: When both birth weight and gestational age of the newborn are available, both should be coded with birth weight sequenced before gestational age.

 Includes: the listed conditions, without further specification, as the cause of morbidity or additional care, in newborn

 Excludes 1: low birth weight due to slow fetal growth and fetal malnutrition (P05.–)

 P07.0 Extremely low birth weight newborn

  Newborn birth weight 999 grams or less

  P07.00 Extremely low birth weight newborn, unspecified weight

  P07.01 Extremely low birth weight newborn, less than 500 grams

  P07.02 Extremely low birth weight newborn, 500–749 grams

  P07.03 Extremely low birth weight newborn, 750–999 grams

 P07.1 Other low birth weight newborn

  Newborn birth weight 1000–2499 grams

  P07.10 Other low birth weight newborn, unspecified weight

  P07.14 Other low birth weight newborn, 1000–1249 grams

  P07.15 Other low birth weight newborn, 1250–1499 grams

  P07.16 Other low birth weight newborn, 1500–1749 grams

  P07.17 Other low birth weight newborn, 1750–1999 grams

  P07.18 Other low birth weight newborn, 2000–2499 grams

Codes P07.2 and P07.3 identify the condition of preterm newborns:

 P07.2 Extreme immaturity of newborn

  Less than 28 completed weeks (less than 196 completed days) of gestation

  P07.20 Extreme immaturity of newborn, unspecified weeks

  P07.21 Extreme immaturity of newborn, less than 24 completed weeks

  P07.22 Extreme immaturity of newborn, 24–26 completed weeks

  P07.23 Extreme immaturity of newborn, 27 completed weeks

 P07.3 Other preterm newborn

  28 completed weeks or more but less than 37 completed weeks (196 completed days but less than 259 completed days) of gestation

  P07.30 Other preterm newborn, unspecified weeks

  P07.31 Other preterm newborn, 28–31 completed weeks

  P07.32 Other preterm newborn, 32–36 completed weeks

Birth Trauma

ICD-9-CM provides just one code for birth trauma. In contrast, an entire block of codes has been designated to describe birth trauma in ICD-10-CM. The codes included in this block are:

Birth trauma (P10–P15)

P10 Intracranial laceration and hemorrhage due to birth injury

P11 Other birth injuries to central nervous system

P12 Birth injury to scalp

P13 Birth injury to skeleton

P14 Birth injury to peripheral nervous system

P15 Other birth injuries

Within each of these codes, greater specificity is afforded at the fourth- and fifth-character levels. For example:

P13   Birth injury to skeleton
    Excludes 2:   birth injury to spine (P11.5)
    P13.0   Fracture of skull due to birth injury
    P13.1   Other birth injuries to skull
        Excludes 1:   cephalhematoma (P12.0)
    P13.2   Birth injury to femur
    P13.3   Birth injury to other long bones
    P13.4   Fracture of clavicle due to birth injury
    P13.8   Birth injuries to other parts of skeleton
    P13.9   Birth injury to skeleton, unspecified

Conditions Assigned to *Other* Categories in ICD-9-CM

Many conditions that are assigned to the *other* categories in ICD-9-CM have been given distinct rubrics in ICD-10-CM. Two examples include neonatal metabolic acidemia and neonatal heart failure.

ICD-9-CM: 768.4   Fetal distress, unspecified as to time of onset in liveborn infant
                       Fetal metabolic acidemia unspecified as to time of onset, in liveborn infant
ICD-10-CM: P19   Metabolic acidemia in newborn

ICD-9-CM: 779.89 Other specified conditions originating in the perinatal period
ICD-10-CM: P29.0   Neonatal cardiac failure

Expansions

A number of codes for conditions originating during the perinatal period have been expanded in ICD-10-CM. For example:

ICD-9-CM: 770.0   Congenital pneumonia
ICD-10-CM: P23   Congenital pneumonia
          P23.0   Congenital pneumonia due to viral agent
          P23.1   Congenital pneumonia due to Chlamydia
          P23.2   Congenital pneumonia due to staphylococcus
          P23.3   Congenital pneumonia due to streptococcus, group B
          P23.4   Congenital pneumonia due to Escherichia coli
          P23.5   Congenital pneumonia due to Pseudomonas
          P23.6   Congenital pneumonia due to other bacterial agents
          P23.8   Congenital pneumonia due to other organisms
                    Use additional code (B97) to identify organism
          P23.9   Congenital pneumonia, unspecified

ICD-9-CM: 770.2   Interstitial emphysema and related conditions
ICD-10-CM: P25   Interstitial emphysema and related conditions originating in the perinatal period
          P25.0   Interstitial emphysema originating in the perinatal period
          P25.1   Pneumothorax originating in the perinatal period
          P25.2   Pneumomediastinum originating in the perinatal period

P25.3 Pneumopericardium originating in the perinatal period
P25.8 Other conditions related to interstitial emphysema originating in the perinatal period

ICD-9-CM: 770.3 Pulmonary hemorrhage
ICD-10-CM: P26 Pulmonary hemorrhage originating in the perinatal period
P26.0 Tracheobronchial hemorrhage originating in the perinatal period
P26.1 Massive pulmonary hemorrhage originating in the perinatal period
P26.8 Other pulmonary hemorrhages originating in the perinatal period
P26.9 Unspecified pulmonary hemorrhage originating in the perinatal period

ICD-9-CM: 772.0 Fetal blood loss
ICD-10-CM: P50 Newborn affected by (intrauterine) blood loss
Excludes 1: congenital anemia from fetal blood loss (P61.3)
P50.0 Newborn affected by fetal (intrauterine) blood loss from vasa previa
P50.1 Newborn affected by fetal blood loss from ruptured cord
P50.2 Newborn affected by fetal blood loss from placenta
P50.3 Newborn affected by hemorrhage into co-twin
P50.4 Newborn affected by hemorrhage into maternal circulation
P50.5 Newborn affected by fetal blood loss from cut end of co-twin's cord
P50.8 Newborn affected by other fetal blood loss
P50.9 Newborn affected by fetal blood loss, unspecified

ICD-9-CM: 772.4 Gastrointestinal hemorrhage
ICD-10-CM: P54 Other neonatal hemorrhages
Excludes 1: newborn affected by (intrauterine) blood loss (P50.–)
pulmonary hemorrhage originating in the perinatal period (P26.–)
P54.0 Neonatal hematemesis
P54.1 Neonatal melena
P54.2 Neonatal rectal hemorrhage
P54.3 Other neonatal gastrointestinal hemorrhage

ICD-9-CM: 774.1 Perinatal jaundice from other excessive hemolysis
ICD-10-CM: P58 Neonatal jaundice due to other excessive hemolysis
Excludes 1: jaundice due to isoimmunization (P55–P57)
P58.0 Neonatal jaundice due to bruising
P58.1 Neonatal jaundice due to bleeding
P58.2 Neonatal jaundice due to infection
P58.3 Neonatal jaundice due to polycythemia
P58.4 Neonatal jaundice due to drugs or toxins transmitted from mother or given to newborn
Code first (T36–T50) to identify drug
P58.41 Neonatal jaundice due to drugs or toxins transmitted from mother
P58.42 Neonatal jaundice due to drugs or toxins given to newborn
P58.5 Neonatal jaundice due to swallowed maternal blood
P58.8 Neonatal jaundice due to other specified excessive hemolysis
P58.9 Neonatal jaundice due to excessive hemolysis, unspecified

ICD-9-CM:	775.5	Other transitory neonatal electrolyte disturbances
ICD-10-CM:	P74	Other transitory neonatal electrolyte and metabolic disturbances

P74.0   Late metabolic acidosis of newborn
P74.1   Dehydration of newborn
P74.2   Disturbances of sodium balance of newborn
P74.3   Disturbances of potassium balance of newborn
P74.4   Other transitory electrolyte disturbances of newborn
P74.5   Transitory tyrosinemia of newborn
P74.6   Transitory hyperammonemia of newborn
P74.8   Other transitory metabolic disturbances of newborn
P74.9   Transitory metabolic disturbance of newborn, unspecified

Because these ICD-10-CM codes provide increased specificity, physicians will need to provide documentation of the specific conditions that affect newborn infants.

Chapter 17

Congenital Malformations, Deformations, and Chromosomal Abnormalities

Chapter 17 of the ICD-10-CM Tabular List classifies congenital malformations, deformations, and chromosomal abnormalities. It includes categories Q00 through Q99, which are arranged in the following blocks:

Q00–Q07   Congenital malformations of the nervous system
Q10–Q18   Congenital malformations of the eye, ear, face and neck
Q20–Q28   Congenital malformations of the circulatory system
Q30–Q34   Congenital malformations of the respiratory system
Q35–Q37   Cleft lip and cleft palate
Q38–Q45   Other congenital malformations of the digestive system
Q50–Q56   Congenital malformations of the genital organs
Q60–Q64   Congenital malformations of the urinary system
Q65–Q79   Congenital malformations and deformations of the musculoskeletal system
Q80–Q89   Other congenital malformations
Q90–Q99   Chromosomal abnormalities, not elsewhere classified

Title Changes

A number of block and category title changes have been made in chapter 17 of ICD-10-CM. A few examples of these changes include the following:

ICD-9-CM: 743.3   Congenital cataract and lens anomalies
ICD-10-CM: Q12   Congenital lens malformations

ICD-9-CM: 743.51   Vitreous anomalies
ICD-10-CM: Q14.0   Congenital malformation of vitreous humor

ICD-9-CM: 758.1   Patau's syndrome
             758.2   Edwards' syndrome
ICD-10-CM: Q91   Trisomy 18 and trisomy 13

Additions, Deletions, and Combinations

When ICD-10-CM chapter 17 is compared with ICD-9-CM chapter 14, Congenital Anomalies, it is evident that many codes have been added, deleted, combined, or moved from one section or chapter to another. For example, conditions that are not assigned specific codes in ICD-9-CM are assigned the following codes in ICD-10-CM:

Q11.3   Macrophthalmos
Q20.6   Isomerism of atrial appendages
Q22.6   Hypoplastic right heart syndrome

Because there is no specific code in ICD-9-CM for peripheral arteriovenous aneurysms, codes have been developed for ICD-10-CM. These codes are classified according to site. For example:

Q27.3   Arteriovenous malformation (peripheral)
    Q27.30   Arteriovenous malformation, site unspecified
    Q27.31   Arteriovenous malformation of vessel of upper limb
    Q27.32   Arteriovenous malformation of vessel of lower limb
    Q27.33   Arteriovenous malformation of digestive system vessel
    Q27.34   Arteriovenous malformation of renal vessel
    Q27.39   Arteriovenous malformation, other site

Expansions

A number of codes for congenital conditions and chromosomal abnormalities have been expanded in ICD-10-CM. For example:

ICD-9-CM: 742.0   Encephalocele
ICD-10-CM: Q01   Encephalocele
    Q01.0   Frontal encephalocele
    Q01.1   Nasofrontal encephalocele
    Q01.2   Occipital encephalocele
    Q01.8   Encephalocele of other sites
    Q01.9   Encephalocele, unspecified

ICD-9-CM: 742.2   Reduction deformities of brain
ICD-10-CM: Q04   Other congenital malformations of brain
    Q04.0   Congenital malformations of corpus callosum
    Q04.1   Arhinencephaly
    Q04.2   Holoprosencephaly
    Q04.3   Other reduction deformities of brain
    Q04.4   Septo-optic dysplasia of brain
    Q04.5   Megalencephaly
    Q04.6   Congenital cerebral cysts
    Q04.8   Other specified congenital malformations of brain
    Q04.9   Congenital malformation of brain, unspecified

ICD-9-CM: 748.1   Other anomalies of nose
ICD-10-CM: Q30   Congenital malformations of nose
    Q30.0   Choanal atresia

Q30.1   Agenesis and underdevelopment of nose
Q30.2   Fissured, notched and cleft nose
Q30.3   Congenital perforated nasal septum
Q30.8   Other congenital malformations of nose
Q30.9   Congenital malformation of nose, unspecified

ICD-9-CM: 748.3   Other anomalies of larynx, trachea, and bronchus
ICD-10-CM: Q31   Congenital malformations of larynx

Q31.0   Web of larynx
Q31.1   Congenital subglottic stenosis
Q31.2   Laryngeal hypoplasia
Q31.3   Laryngocele
Q31.4   Congenital laryngeal stridor
Q31.8   Other congenital malformations of larynx
Q31.9   Congenital malformation of larynx, unspecified

ICD-9-CM: 749.0   Cleft palate

749.00   Cleft palate, unspecified
749.01   Unilateral, complete
749.02   Unilateral, incomplete
749.03   Bilateral, complete
749.04   Bilateral, incomplete

ICD-10-CM: Q35   Cleft palate

Q35.1   Cleft hard palate
Q35.3   Cleft soft palate
Q35.5   Cleft hard palate with cleft soft palate
Q35.6   Cleft palate, medial
Q35.7   Cleft uvula
Q35.9   Cleft palate, unspecified

ICD-9-CM: 750.3   Tracheoesophageal fistula, esophageal atresia and stenosis
ICD-10-CM: Q39   Congenital malformations of esophagus

Q39.0   Atresia of esophagus without fistula
Q39.1   Atresia of esophagus with tracheo-esophageal fistula
Q39.2   Congenital tracheo-esophageal fistula without atresia
Q39.3   Congenital stenosis and stricture of esophagus
Q39.4   Esophageal web
Q39.5   Congenital dilatation of esophagus
Q39.6   Congenital diverticulum of esophagus
Q39.8   Other congenital malformations of esophagus
Q39.9   Congenital malformation of esophagus, unspecified

ICD-9-CM: 752.61   Hypospadias
ICD-10-CM: Q54   Hypospadias

Q54.0   Hypospadias, balanic
Q54.1   Hypospadias, penile
Q54.2   Hypospadias, penoscrotal
Q54.3   Hypospasias, perineal
Q54.4   Congenital chordee
Q54.8   Other hypospadias
Q54.9   Hypospadias, unspecified

ICD-9-CM: 757.6   Specified anomalies of breast
ICD-10-CM: Q83   Congenital malformations of breast
                        Q83.0   Congenital absence of breast with absent nipple
                        Q83.1   Accessory breast
                        Q83.2   Absent nipple
                        Q83.3   Accessory nipple
                        Q83.8   Other congenital malformations of breast
                        Q83.9   Congenital malformation of breast, unspecified

As with many other chapters in ICD-10-CM, laterality is identified at the fourth- or fifth-character level in chapter 17. For example:

Q53   Undescended and ectopic testicle
        Q53.0   Ectopic testis
                Q53.00   Ectopic testis, unspecified
                Q53.01   Ectopic testis, unilateral
                Q53.02   Ectopic testes, bilateral

Q65   Congenital deformities of hip
        Q65.0   Congenital dislocation of hip, unilateral
                Q65.00   Congenital dislocation of hip, unilateral, unspecified side
                Q65.01   Congenital dislocation of right hip
                Q65.02   Congenital dislocation of left hip
        Q65.1   Congenital dislocation of hip, bilateral
        Q65.2   Congenital dislocation of hip, unspecified
        Q65.3   Congenital partial dislocation of hip, unilateral
                Q65.30   Congenital partial dislocation of hip, unilateral, unspecified side
                Q65.31   Congenital partial dislocation of right hip
                Q65.32   Congenital partial dislocation of left hip
        Q65.4   Congenital partial dislocation of hip, bilateral
        Q65.5   Congenital partial dislocation of hip, unspecified
        Q65.6   Congenital unstable hip
        Q65.8   Other congenital deformities of hip
        Q65.9   Congenital deformity of hip, unspecified

Reduction Defects of Upper and Lower Limbs

In ICD-10-CM, the codes to identify reduction defects of the upper and lower limbs have changed significantly from ICD-9-CM in relation to format and terminology. The codes again use fourth and fifth characters to identify the laterality of the defect. For example:

Q71   Reduction defects of upper limb
        Q71.0   Congenital complete absence of upper limb
                Q71.00   Congenital complete absence of upper limb, unspecified side
                Q71.01   Congenital complete absence of right upper limb
                Q71.02   Congenital complete absence of left upper limb
                Q71.03   Congenital complete absence of upper limb, bilateral
        Q71.6   Lobster-claw hand
                Q71.60   Lobster-claw hand, unspecified side
                Q71.61   Lobster-claw right hand
                Q71.62   Lobster-claw left hand
                Q71.63   Lobster-claw hand, bilateral

Q72   Reduction defects of lower limb
    Q72.4   Longitudinal reduction defect of femur
        Q72.40   Longitudinal reduction defect of femur, unspecified side
        Q72.41   Longitudinal reduction defect of right femur
        Q72.42   Longitudinal defect of left femur
        Q72.43   Longitudinal defect of femur, bilateral

Chromosomal Anomalies

In ICD-9-CM, category 758 is used to report chromosomal anomalies. In ICD-10-CM, several blocks of codes are assigned to reporting chromosomal abnormalities.

Chromosomal abnormalities, not elsewhere classified (Q90–Q99)
Q90   Down syndrome
Q91   Trisomy 18 and trisomy 13
Q92   Other trisomies and partial trisomies of the autosomes, not elsewhere classified
Q93   Monosomies and deletions from the autosomes, not elsewhere classified
Q95   Balanced rearrangements and structural markers, not elsewhere classified
Q96   Turner syndrome
Q97   Other sex chromosome abnormalities, female phenotype, not elsewhere classified
Q98   Other sex chromosome abnormalities, male phenotype, not elsewhere classified
Q99   Other chromosome abnormalities, not elsewhere classified

Some examples of codes in this block include:

Q91   Trisomy 18 and trisomy 13
    Q91.0   Trisomy 18, nonmosaicism (meiotic nondisjunction)
    Q91.1   Trisomy 18, mosaicism (mitotic nondisjunction)
    Q91.2   Trisomy 18, translocation
    Q91.3   Trisomy 18, unspecified
    Q91.4   Trisomy 13, nonmosaicism (meiotic nondisjunction)
    Q91.5   Trisomy 13, mosaicism (mitotic nondisjunction)
    Q91.6   Trisomy 13, translocation
    Q91.7   Trisomy 13, unspecified

Q96   Turner syndrome
    Q96.0   Karyotype 45, X
    Q96.1   Karyotype 46, X iso(Xq)
    Q96.2   Karyotype 46, X with abnormal sex chromosome, except iso(Xq)
    Q96.3   Mosaicism, 45, X/46, XX or XY
    Q96.4   Mosaicism, 45, X/other cell line(s) with abnormal sex chromosome
    Q96.8   Other variants of Turner syndrome
    Q96.9   Turner syndrome, unspecified

Chapter 18

Symptoms, Signs, and Abnormal Clinical and Laboratory Findings, Not Elsewhere Classified

Chapter 18 classifies symptoms, signs, and abnormal clinical and laboratory findings that are not classified elsewhere in the ICD-10-CM Tabular List. It includes categories R00 through R99, which are arranged in the following blocks:

R00–R09   Symptoms and signs involving the circulatory and respiratory systems
R10–R19   Symptoms and signs involving the digestive system and abdomen
R20–R23   Symptoms and signs involving the skin and subcutaneous tissue
R25–R29   Symptoms and signs involving the nervous and musculoskeletal systems
R30–R39   Symptoms and signs involving the urinary system
R40–R46   Symptoms and signs involving cognition, perception, emotional state and behavior
R47–R49   Symptoms and signs involving speech and voice
R50–R69   General symptoms and signs
R70–R79   Abnormal findings on examination of blood, without diagnosis
R80–R82   Abnormal findings on examination of urine, without diagnosis
R83–R89   Abnormal findings on examination of other body fluids, substances and tissues, without diagnosis
R90–R94   Abnormal findings on diagnostic imaging and in function studies, without diagnosis
R99   Ill-defined and unknown cause of mortality

Chapter 18 includes codes for symptoms, signs, abnormal results of clinical or other investigative procedures, and ill-defined conditions that are assigned when no diagnosis was made that can be classified elsewhere. Signs and symptoms that point to a given, established diagnosis are assigned to other chapters in the classification system. The categories in this chapter include less well defined conditions and symptoms. The many *excludes* statements that accompany the codes in this chapter serve to remind users that other codes may be more appropriate.

Title Changes

A number of block and category title changes have been made in chapter 18 of ICD-10-CM. A few examples of these changes include the following:

ICD-9-CM: 786   Symptoms involving respiratory system and other chest symptoms
ICD-10-CM: R06   Abnormalities of breathing

ICD-9-CM: 789   Other symptoms involving abdomen and pelvis
ICD-10-CM: R19   Other symptoms and signs involving the digestive system and abdomen

Additions, Deletions, and Combinations

When chapter 18 of ICD-10-CM is compared with chapter 16, Symptoms, Signs, and Ill-Defined Conditions, of ICD-9-CM, it is evident that many codes have been added, deleted, combined, or moved from one section or chapter to another. Bradycardia, pleurisy, dry mouth, elevated white blood count, and pancytopenia are examples of conditions that are assigned to chapter 18 of ICD-10-CM.

ICD-9-CM: 427.89   Other specified cardiac dysrhythmias
ICD-10-CM: R00.1   Bradycardia, unspecified

ICD-9-CM: 511.0   Pleurisy without mention of effusion or current tuberculosis
ICD-10-CM: R09.1   Pleurisy

ICD-9-CM: 527.7   Disturbance of salivary secretion
ICD-10-CM: R68.2   Dry mouth, unspecified

ICD-9-CM: 288.8   Other specified disease of white blood cells
ICD-10-CM: R72.0   Elevated white blood cell count

ICD-9-CM: 284.8   Other specified aplastic anemia
ICD-10-CM: R79.1   Pancytopenia

Several conditions classified to ICD-10-CM categories and codes are not included as specific ICD-9-CM codes. Some examples include the following:

R33.0   Drug induced retention of urine
       Code first (T36–T50) to identify the drug

R46   Symptoms and signs involving appearance and behavior
       Excludes 1:   appearance and behavior in schizophrenia, schizotypal and delusional
                   disorders (F20–F29)
                   mental and behavioral disorders (F01–F99)
       R46.0   Very low level of personal hygiene
       R46.1   Bizarre personal appearance
       R46.2   Strange and inexplicable behavior
       R46.3   Overactivity
       R46.4   Slowness and poor responsiveness
       R46.5   Suspiciousness and marked evasiveness
       R46.6   Undue concern and preoccupation with stressful events
       R46.7   Verbosity and circumstantial detail obscuring reason for contact
       R46.8   Other symptoms and signs involving appearance and behavior
              R46.81   Obsessive-compulsive behavior
              R46.89   Other symptoms and signs involving appearance and behavior

R58   Hemorrhage, not elsewhere classified

R77   Other abnormalities of plasma proteins
      R77.0   Abnormality of albumin
      R77.1   Abnormality of globulin
      R77.2   Abnormality of alphafetoprotein
      R77.8   Other specified abnormalities of plasma proteins
      R77.9   Abnormality of plasma protein, unspecified

R78   Findings of drugs and other substances, not normally found in blood
      Excludes 1:   mental or behavioral disorders due to psychoactive substance use
                (F10–F19)
      R78.0   Finding of alcohol in blood
           Use additional external cause code (Y90.–) for detail regarding
             alcohol level
      R78.1   Finding of opiate drug in blood
      R78.2   Finding of cocaine in blood
      R78.3   Finding of hallucinogen in blood
      R78.4   Finding of other drugs of addictive potential in blood
      R78.5   Finding of other psychotropic drug in blood
      R78.6   Finding of steroid agent in blood
      R78.7   Finding of abnormal level of heavy metals in blood
      R78.8   Finding of other specified substances, not normally found in blood
            R78.81   Bacteremia
            R78.89   Finding of other specified substances, not normally found in blood
      R78.9   Finding of unspecified substance, not normally found in blood

Expansions

A number of codes for symptoms, signs, and abnormal clinical and laboratory findings have been expanded in ICD-10-CM.

Expansions to Fourth- and Fifth-Character Levels

In several instances, codes have been expanded at the fourth- and fifth-character levels to add specificity. For example:

ICD-9-CM: 787.3   Flatulence, eructation and gas pain
ICD-10-CM: R14   Flatulence and related conditions
                   R14.0   Abdominal distension (gaseous)
                   R14.1   Gas pain
                   R14.2   Eructation
                   R14.3   Flatulence
                   R14.8   Other

ICD-9-CM: 782.0   Disturbance of skin sensation
ICD-10-CM: R20   Disturbances of skin sensation
                   R20.0   Anesthesia of skin
                   R20.1   Hypoesthesia of skin
                   R20.2   Paresthesia of skin
                   R20.3   Hyperesthesia
                   R20.8   Other disturbances of skin sensation
                   R20.9   Unspecified disturbance of skin sensation

| ICD-9-CM: | 781.2 | Abnormality of gait |
| ICD-10-CM: | R26 | Abnormalities of gait and mobility |

     R26.0 Ataxic gait
     R26.1 Paralytic gait
     R26.2 Difficulty in walking, not elsewhere classified
     R26.8 Other abnormalities of gait and mobility
          R26.81 Falling
          R26.82 Unsteadiness on feet
          R26.89 Other abnormalities of gait and mobility
     R26.9 Unspecified abnormalities of gait and mobility

| ICD-9-CM: | 781.1 | Disturbances of smell and taste |
| ICD-10-CM: | R43 | Disturbances of smell and taste |

     R43.0 Anosmia
     R43.1 Parosmia
     R43.2 Parageusia
     R43.8 Other disturbances of smell and taste
     R43.9 Unspecified disturbances of smell and taste

| ICD-9-CM: | 780.99 | Generalized pain |
| ICD-10-CM: | R52 | Pain, not elsewhere classified |

     R52.0 Acute pain
          R52.00 Acute pain, unspecified
          R52.01 Acute postoperative pain
          R52.02 Acute pain in neoplastic disease
          R52.09 Other acute pain
     R52.1 Chronic intractable pain
          R52.10 Chronic intractable pain, unspecified
          R52.11 Chronic intractable postoperative pain
          R52.12 Chronic intractable pain in neoplastic disease
          R52.19 Other chronic intractable pain
     R52.2 Other chronic pain
          R52.20 Other chronic pain, unspecified
          R52.21 Other chronic postoperative pain
          R52.22 Other chronic pain in neoplastic disease
          R52.29 Other chronic pain
     R52.9 Pain, unspecified

Abnormal Findings

All the codes in the blocks on abnormal findings on examination of other body fluids, substances, and tissues, without diagnosis (R83–R89), have been significantly expanded to provide greater specificity. The codes within this block include:

R83   Abnormal findings in cerebrospinal fluid
R84   Abnormal findings in specimens from respiratory organs and thorax
R85   Abnormal findings in specimens from digestive organs and abdominal cavity
R86   Abnormal findings in specimens from male genital organs
R87   Abnormal findings in specimens from female genital organs
R88   Abnormal findings in other body fluids and substances
R89   Abnormal findings in specimens from other organs, systems and tissues

The following example shows the increased specificity available with category R83:

R83 Abnormal findings in cerebrospinal fluid
    R83.0 Abnormal level of enzymes in cerebrospinal fluid
    R83.2 Abnormal level of other drugs, medicaments and biological substances in cerebrospinal fluid
    R83.3 Abnormal level of substances chiefly nonmedicinal as to source in cerebrospinal fluid
    R83.4 Abnormal immunological findings in cerebrospinal fluid
    R83.5 Abnormal microbiological findings in cerebrospinal fluid
    R83.6 Abnormal cytological findings in cerebrospinal fluid
    R83.7 Abnormal histological findings in cerebrospinal fluid
    R83.8 Other abnormal findings in cerebrospinal fluid
    R83.9 Unspecified abnormal finding in cerebrospinal fluid

Each of the codes in this block has similar specificity at the fourth-character level.

Coma

There are significant changes in the coding of coma in ICD-10-CM. In ICD-9-CM, the correct code for coma is 780.01 with no additional specificity. ICD-10-CM provides codes to classify the condition in more detail. Thus, it follows that physicians will need to take greater care in documenting the characteristics of a patient's coma. According to the coding guidelines for ICD-10-CM, the Glascow coma scale must be used in conjunction with the codes for traumatic brain injuries or the sequelae of cerebrovascular accidents. With code R40.2–, one code from each of the three subcategories must be assigned to complete the Glascow scale. When more than one coma assessment is performed, the patient's health record should include a report of the initial coma scale performed at the time of admission and a final rating performed at the time of discharge. Facility policy should determine which scale ratings are to be reported in the health record. An extension must be added to the coma codes to indicate which ratings are to be reported in the final record.

R40.2 Coma
Coma NOS
Unconsciousness NOS
Code first any associated:
    coma in skull fracture (S02.–)
    coma in intracranial injury (S06.–)
The following 7th character extensions are to be added to codes R40.21, R40.22, R40.23:
1 in the field [EMT or ambulance]
2 at arrival to emergency department
3 at hospital admission
4 24 hours after hospital admission
9 unspecified time
A code from each subcategory is required to complete the coma scale
Note: These codes are intended primarily for trauma registry and research use but may be utilized by all users of the classification who wish to collect this information.
R40.20 Unspecified coma
R40.21 Coma scale, eyes open
    R40.211 Coma scale, eyes open, never
    R40.212 Coma scale, eyes open, to pain
    R40.213 Coma scale, eyes open, to sound
    R40.214 Coma scale, eyes open, spontaneous

R40.22   Coma scale, best verbal response
    R40.221   Coma scale, best verbal response, none
    R40.222   Coma scale, best verbal response, incomprehensible words
    R40.223   Coma scale, best verbal response, inappropriate words
    R40.224   Coma scale, best verbal response, confused conversation
    R40.225   Coma scale, best verbal response, oriented
R40.23   Coma scale, best motor response
    R40.231   Coma scale, best motor response, none
    R40.232   Coma scale, best motor response, extension
    R40.233   Coma scale, best motor response, abnormal
    R40.234   Coma scale, best motor response, flexion withdrawal
    R40.235   Coma scale, best motor response, localizes pain
    R40.236   Coma scale, best motor response, obeys commands

Chapter 19

Injury, Poisoning, and Other Consequences of External Causes

Chapter 19 of the ICD-10-CM Tabular List classifies injuries, poisonings, and certain other consequences resulting from external factors. It includes categories S00 through T88, which are arranged in the following blocks:

S00–S09 Injuries to the head

S10–S19 Injuries to the neck

S20–S29 Injuries to the thorax

S30–S39 Injuries to the abdomen, lower back, lumbar spine, pelvis and external genitals

S40–S49 Injuries to the shoulder and upper arm

S50–S59 Injuries to the elbow and forearm

S60–S69 Injuries to the wrist and hand

S70–S79 Injuries to the hip and thigh

S80–S89 Injuries to the knee and lower leg

S90–S99 Injuries to the ankle and foot

T07 Unspecified multiple injuries

T14 Injury of unspecified body region

T15–T19 Effects of foreign body entering through natural orifice

T20–T32 Burns and corrosions

T33–T34 Frostbite

T36–T50 Poisoning by, adverse effect of and underdosing of drugs, medicaments and biological substances

T51–T65 Toxic effects of substances chiefly nonmedicinal as to source

T66–T78 Other and unspecified effects of external causes

T79 Certain early complications of trauma

T80–T88 Complications of surgical and medical care, not elsewhere classified

Coding professionals will need to depend heavily on documentation in order to completely and accurately code diagnoses from chapter 19. X-ray reports will be an important tool to use in selecting the correct codes.

The codes in this chapter provide very specific information. For example:

S66.42 Laceration of intrinsic muscle and tendon of thumb at wrist and hand level

S72.021 Displaced fracture of epiphysis (separation) (upper) of right femur

S72.461   Displaced supracondylar fracture with intracondylar extension of lower end of right femur

S75.221   Major laceration of greater saphenous vein at hip and thigh level, right leg

S79.121   Salter-Harris type II physeal fracture of lower end of right femur

S95.211   Laceration of dorsal vein of right foot

Additions, Deletions, and Combinations

When chapter 19 of ICD-10-CM is compared with chapter 17, Injury and Poisoning, of ICD-9-CM, it is evident that many codes have been added, deleted, combined, or moved from one section or chapter to another.

The S section of ICD-10-CM chapter 19 provides codes for the various types of injuries related to single body regions. The T section covers injuries to unspecified body regions as well as poisonings and certain other consequences of external causes. The S section's format is a departure from ICD-9-CM coding in that the blocks cover single body regions, with category codes within each block representing various types of injuries or specific anatomical parts. For example:

Injuries to the head (S00–S09)
S00   Superficial injury of head
S01   Open wound of head
S02   Fracture of skull and facial bones
S03   Dislocation and sprain of joints and ligaments of head
S04   Injury of cranial nerve
S05   Injury of eye and orbit
S06   Intracranial injury
S07   Crushing injury of head
S08   Avulsion and traumatic amputation of part of head
S09   Other and unspecified injuries of head

All the blocks in the S section follow a similar format. In addition, at the beginning of many of the blocks, an *includes* note identifies structures included in that block. For example:

Injuries to the thorax (S20–S29)
Includes: injuries of breast
injuries of chest (wall)
injuries of interscapular area

Injuries to the abdomen, lower back, lumbar spine, pelvis and external genitals (S30–S39)
Includes: injuries to the abdominal wall
injuries to the anus
injuries to the buttock
injuries to the external genitalia
injuries to the flank
injuries to the groin

ICD-10-CM does not provide a specific code for nonhealing surgical wounds (ICD-9-CM code 998.83). In ICD-10-CM, this condition is reported with code T81.89, Other complications of procedures, not elsewhere classified.

Expansions

A number of codes for injuries, poisonings, and other consequences of external causes have been expanded in ICD-10-CM.

Use of Extensions

Extensions are used in most of the codes in chapter 19 and occupy the final-character position. Many of the codes use the following extensions:

a   initial encounter
d   subsequent encounter
q   sequela

Codes in ICD-10 that refer to late effects have been deactivated in ICD-10-CM and replaced with the extension q. Some codes have unique extensions. For example:

S32   Fracture of lumbar spine and pelvis
     A fracture not identified as displaced or nondisplaced should be coded to displaced
     Includes: fracture of lumbosacral neural arch
                fracture of lumbosacral spinous process
                fracture of lumbosacral transverse process
                fracture of lumbosacral vertebra
                fracture of lumbosacral vertebral arch
     Code first any associated spinal cord and spinal nerve injury (S34.–)

A fracture not identified as opened or closed should be coded to closed
The following 7th character extensions are to be added to each code for this category:
    a   initial encounter for closed fracture
    b   initial encounter for open fracture
    d   subsequent encounter for fracture with routine healing
    g   subsequent encounter for fracture with delayed healing
    j   subsequent encounter for fracture with nonunion
    q   sequela

Identification of Laterality

Laterality in ICD-10-CM is identified at the fourth-, fifth-, or sixth-character level. For example:

S40   Superficial injury of shoulder and upper arm
     S40.0   Contusion of shoulder and upper arm
          S40.01   Contusion of shoulder
                 S40.011   Contusion of right shoulder
                 S40.012   Contusion of left shoulder
                 S40.019   Contusion of shoulder, unspecified side

S62.1   Fracture of other and unspecified carpal bone(s)
     S62.10   Fracture of unspecified carpal bone
              S62.101   Fracture of unspecified carpal bone, right wrist
              S62.102   Fracture of unspecified carpal bone, left wrist
              S62.109   Fracture of unspecified carpal bone, unspecified wrist

Associated Injuries

Chapter 19, like many others in ICD-10-CM, directs users to code associated injuries. For example:

S21   Open wound of thorax
       Code also any associated injury (to) (such as):
           heart (S26.–)
           intrathoracic organs (S27.–)
           rib fracture (S22.3–, S22.4–)
           spinal cord injury (S24.0–, S24.1–)
           traumatic hemothorax (S27.1)
           traumatic hemopneumothorax (S27.3)
           traumatic pneumothorax (S27.0)
           wound infection

Codes related to poisonings and certain other consequences of external causes are found in T07 through T88. Categories T00 through T06 and T08 through T13 have been deactivated in ICD-10-CM. Category T07, Unspecified multiple injuries, is used only when no documentation is available to identify the specific injuries. This code would not be used in the inpatient setting. Category T14, Injury of unspecified body region, is used only when no documentation is available to identify the specific injury. Like T07, this category is not intended for use in the inpatient setting.

Categories T15 through T19, Effects of foreign body entering through natural orifice, identify the presence of a foreign body in a body region. For example, T15 identifies foreign body on external eye. These codes require extension codes to identify whether the visit is the initial encounter, a subsequent encounter, or a sequela. These codes are generally the same as in ICD-9-CM. Laterality is incorporated into the codes at the fifth-character level. For example:

T15.0   Foreign body in cornea
         T15.00   Foreign body in cornea, unspecified eye
         T15.01   Foreign body in cornea, right eye
         T15.02   Foreign body in cornea, left eye
T15.1   Foreign body in conjunctival sac
         T15.10   Foreign body in conjunctival sac, unspecified eye
         T15.11   Foreign body in conjunctival sac, right eye
         T15.12   Foreign body in conjunctival sac, left eye

Burns and Corrosions

Codes from block T20 through T32 identify burns and corrosions in ICD-10-CM. The addition of the term *corrosion* is new in ICD-10-CM. The block includes various codes that first identify the anatomic site of the burns, and then fourth and fifth characters identify the degree of the burn. For example:

T21   Burn and corrosion of trunk
       Includes: Burns and corrosion of hip region
       Excludes 2:   burns and corrosion of:
                           axilla (T22.– with fifth character 4)
                           scapular region (T22.– with fifth character 6)
                           shoulder (T22.– with fifth character 5)
       T21.0   Burn of unspecified degree of trunk
       T21.1   Burn of first degree of trunk
                T21.10   Burn of first degree of trunk, unspecified site
                T21.11   Burn of first degree of chest wall

T21.12   Burn of first degree of abdominal wall
T21.13   Burn of first degree of upper back
T21.14   Burn of first degree of lower back
T21.15   Burn of first degree of buttock
T21.16   Burn of first degree of male genital region
T21.17   Burn of first degree of female genital region
T21.19   Burn of first degree of other site of trunk

The other fourth-character subcategory codes include the following:

T21.2   Burn of second degree of trunk
T21.3   Burn of third degree of trunk
T21.4   Corrosion of unspecified degree of trunk
T21.5   Corrosion of first degree of trunk
T21.6   Corrosion of second degree of trunk
T21.7   Corrosion of third degree of trunk

All the codes for burns direct users to code an additional external cause code to identify the source, place, and intent of the burn. The codes for corrosions direct the user to code first the chemical and intent and to use an additional code to identify the place.

Frostbite

The codes for frostbite have been expanded from one code in ICD-9-CM into two in ICD-10-CM: T33, Superficial frostbite, and T34, Frostbite with tissue necrosis. Fourth and fifth characters identify the specific sites of the frostbite. For example:

T33   Superficial frostbite
    T33.0   Superficial frostbite of head
        T33.01   Superficial frostbite of ear
            T33.011   Superficial frostbite of right ear
            T33.012   Superficial frostbite of left ear
            T33.019   Superficial frostbite of unspecified ear
        T33.02   Superficial frostbite of nose
        T33.09   Superficial frostbite of other part of head

Poisonings versus Adverse Effects

ICD-10-CM does not provide different category codes to identify poisonings versus adverse effects. The various codes in T36 through T50 (Poisoning by, adverse effects of and underdosing of drugs, medicaments and biological substances) identify the substances causing the adverse effect. In addition, fifth and sixth characters indicate the circumstances that caused the adverse effect, such as accidental poisoning or adverse effect, intentional self-harm, assault, or undetermined cause. For example:

T36   Poisoning by, adverse effect of and underdosing of systemic antibiotics
    Excludes 1:   antineoplastic antibiotics (T45.1)
                 locally applied antibiotic NEC (T49.0)
                 topically used antibiotic for ear, nose and throat (T49.6)
                 topically used antibiotic for eye (T49.5)

The following extensions are to be added to each code for category T36:
a   initial encounter
d   subsequent encounter
q   sequela

T36.0   Poisoning by and adverse effect of penicillins

     T36.0x   Poisoning by and adverse effect of penicillins

          T36.0x1   Poisoning by penicillins, accidental (unintentional)

          T36.0x2   Poisoning by penicillins, intentional self-harm

          T36.0x3   Poisoning by penicillins, assault

          T36.0x4   Poisoning by penicillins, undetermined

          T36.0x5   Adverse effect of penicillins

          T36.0x6   Underdosing of penicillins

The user is directed to code to accidental poisoning when no intent of poisoning is indicated. Undetermined intent is only for use when there is specific documentation in the record that the intent of the injury cannot be determined.

Other fourth-character subclassification codes in category T36, Poisonings by and adverse effect of systemic antibiotics, identify poisonings with and adverse effects of cephalosporins, chloramphenicol group, macrolides, tetracyclines, aminoglycosides, rifampicins, antifungal antibiotics, and other systemic antibiotics.

Other codes in this block include codes for poisonings and adverse effects of the following medications:

- Other systemic and antiinfectives and antiparasitics (T37)

- Hormones (T38)

- Nonopioid analgesics, antipyretics, and antirheumatics (T39)

- Narcotics and psychodysleptics (T40)

- Anesthetics and therapeutic gases (T41)

- Antiepileptic, sedative hypnotic, and antiparkinsonism drugs (T42)

- Psychotropic drugs (T43)

- Drugs affecting the autonomic nervous system (T44)

- Hematological agents (T45)

- Drugs affecting the cardiovascular system (T46)

- Drugs affecting the gastrointestinal system (T47)

- Drugs affecting the smooth and skeletal muscles and the respiratory system (T48)

- Topical agents affecting the skin and mucous membrane and ophthalmological, otorhinolaryngological, and dental drugs (T49)

- Diuretics (T50)

Toxic Substances

Contact with toxic substances or exposure to toxic substances is reported using codes from T51 through T65, Toxic effects of substances chiefly nonmedicinal as to source. Users are reminded to use an additional code or codes for all associated manifestations of toxic effect such as respiratory conditions due to external agents (J60–J70). Categories within this block include the following:

T51   Toxic effect of alcohol
T52   Toxic effect of organic solvents
T53   Toxic effect of halogen derivatives of aliphatic and aromatic hydrocarbons
T54   Toxic effect of corrosive substances
T55   Toxic effect of soaps and detergents
T56   Toxic effect of metals
T57   Toxic effect of other inorganic substances
T58   Toxic effect of carbon monoxide
T59   Toxic effect of other gases, fumes and vapors
T60   Toxic effect of pesticides
T61   Toxic effect of noxious substances eaten as seafood
T62   Toxic effect of other noxious substances eaten as food
T63   Toxic effect of contact with venomous animals and plants
T64   Toxic effect of aflatoxin and other mycotoxin food contaminants
T65   Toxic effect of other and unspecified substances

Fourth characters specify the particular product. For example, the fourth characters for T52, Toxic effect of organic solvents, include:

T52.0   Toxic effects of petroleum products
T52.1   Toxic effects of benzene
T52.2   Toxic effects of homologues of benzene
T52.3   Toxic effects of glycols
T52.4   Toxic effects of ketones
T52.8   Toxic effects of other organic solvents
T52.9   Toxic effects of unspecified organic solvent

Fifth and sixth characters identify the intent (accidental, self-harm, assault, or undetermined) of the poisoning. For example:

T52.1   Toxic effects of benzene
    T52.1x   Toxic effects of benzene
        T52.1x1   Toxic effect of benzene, accidental (unintentional)
        T52.1x2   Toxic effect of benzene, intentional self-harm
        T52.1x3   Toxic effect of benzene, assault
        T52.1x4   Toxic effect of benzene, undetermined

Extensions are used to indicate whether the visit is for the initial encounter, subsequent encounter, or sequela of the toxic effect.

Effects of External Causes

T66 through T78, Other and unspecified effects of external causes, include the following category codes:

T66   Unspecified effects of radiation
T67   Effects of heat and light
T68   Hypothermia
T69   Other effects of reduced temperature
T70   Effects of pressure and water pressure
T71   Asphyxiation

T73   Effects of other deprivation

T74   Adult and child abuse, neglect and other maltreatment, confirmed

T75   Other and unspecified effects of other external causes

T76   Adult and child abuse, neglect and other maltreatment, suspected

T78   Adverse effects, not elsewhere classified

These categories are very similar to ICD-9-CM but provide added specificity. For example:

ICD-9-CM: 994.7   Asphyxiation and strangulation
ICD-10-CM: T71.1   Asphyxiation due to mechanical threat to breathing
             T71.2   Asphyxiation due to systemic oxygen deficiency due to low oxygen content in ambient air
             T71.9   Asphyxiation due to unspecified cause

Subcategory codes T71.1 and T71.2 include several fifth and sixth characters. For example:

T71.22   Asphyxiation due to being trapped in a car trunk
      T71.221   Asphyxiation due to being trapped in a car trunk, accidental
      T71.222   Asphyxiation due to being trapped in a car trunk, intentional self-harm
      T71.223   Asphyxiation due to being trapped in a car trunk, assault
      T71.224   Asphyxiation due to being trapped in a car trunk, undetermined

Early Complications of Trauma

Category code T79, Certain early complications of trauma, not elsewhere classified, includes fourth-character subclassification codes for the following conditions:

T79.0   Air embolism (traumatic)

T79.1   Fat embolism (traumatic)

T79.2   Traumatic secondary and recurrent hemorrhage

T79.4   Traumatic shock

T79.5   Traumatic anuria

T79.6   Traumatic ischemia of muscle

T79.7   Traumatic subcutaneous emphysema

T79.8   Other early complications of trauma

T79.9   Unspecified early complications of trauma

Use of Additional External Cause Codes

For codes from T80 through T88, Complications of surgical and medical care, not elsewhere classified, users are advised to use an additional external cause code to identify devices involved and details of circumstances. These ICD-10-CM codes are very similar to ICD-9-CM codes but offer greater specificity. For example:

ICD-9-CM: 998.4   Foreign body accidentally left during a procedure
ICD-10-CM: T81.5   Complications of foreign body accidentally left in body following procedure
             T81.50   Unspecified complication of foreign body accidentally left in body following procedure
             T81.51   Adhesions due to foreign body accidentally left in body following procedure

T81.52   Obstruction due to foreign body accidentally left in body
          following procedure
T81.53   Perforation due to foreign body accidentally left in body
          following procedure
T81.59   Other complications of foreign body accidentally left in body
          following procedure

Each of these fifth-character subclassifications is divided into sixth characters to reflect the type of procedure during which the foreign body was left. For example:

T81.51   Adhesions due to foreign body accidentally left in body following
          procedure
          T81.510   Adhesions due to foreign body accidentally left in body following surgical
                     operation
          T81.511   Adhesions due to foreign body accidentally left in body following infusion
                     or transfusion
          T81.512   Adhesions due to foreign body accidentally left in body following kidney
                     dialysis
          T81.513   Adhesions due to foreign body accidentally left in body following injection
                     or immunization
          T81.514   Adhesions due to foreign body accidentally left in body following
                     endoscopic examination
          T81.515   Adhesions due to foreign body accidentally left in body following heart
                     catheterization
          T81.516   Adhesions due to foreign body accidentally left in body following aspiration,
                     puncture or other catheterization
          T81.517   Adhesions due to foreign body accidentally left in body following removal
                     of catheter or packing
          T81.518   Adhesions due to foreign body accidentally left in body following other
                     procedure
          T81.519   Adhesions due to foreign body accidentally left in body following
                     unspecified procedure

Mechanical Complications

The number of codes available in ICD-10-CM to code mechanical complications has increased dramatically. For example:

ICD-9-CM: 996.54   Mechanical complication due to breast prosthesis
ICD-10-CM: T85.4   Mechanical complication of breast prosthesis and implant
             T85.41   Breakdown (mechanical) of breast prosthesis and implant
             T85.42   Displacement of breast prosthesis and implant
             T85.43   Leakage of breast prosthesis and implant
             T85.49   Other mechanical complication of breast prosthesis and
                       implant

A similar format is used for the reporting of infections and inflammatory reactions to internal prostheses or implants. For example:

T84.5   Infection and inflammatory reaction due to internal joint prosthesis
         Use additional code to identify infection
         T84.50   Infection and inflammatory reaction due to unspecified internal joint prosthesis
         T84.51   Infection and inflammatory reaction due to internal right hip prosthesis

T84.52   Infection and inflammatory reaction due to internal left hip prosthesis

T84.53   Infection and inflammatory reaction due to internal right knee prosthesis

T84.54   Infection and inflammatory reaction due to internal left knee prosthesis

T84.59   Infection and inflammatory reaction due to other internal joint prosthesis

Other examples of codes for complications include:

T86   Complications of transplanted organs and tissue
    T86.0   Complications of bone-marrow transplant
        T86.00   Unspecified complication of bone-marrow transplant
        T86.01   Graft-versus-host reaction or disease
        T86.09   Other complications of bone-marrow transplant

T87   Complications peculiar to reattachment and amputation
    T87.0   Complications of reattached (part of) upper extremity
        T87.0x   Complications of reattached (part of) upper extremity
            T87.0x1   Complications of reattached (part of) right upper extremity
            T87.0x2   Complications of reattached (part of) left upper extremity
            T87.0xq   Complications of reattached (part of) upper extremity, unspecified side

T88   Other complications of surgical and medical care, not elsewhere classified
    T88.0   Infection following immunization
    T88.1   Other complications following immunization, not elsewhere classified
    T88.2   Shock due to anesthesia
    T88.3   Malignant hyperthermia due to anesthesia
    T88.4   Failed or difficult intubation
    T88.5   Other complications of anesthesia
        T88.51   Hypothermia following anesthesia
        T88.52   Other complications of anesthesia
    T88.6   Anaphylactic shock due to adverse effect of correct drug or medicament substance properly administered
    T88.7   Unspecified adverse effect of drug or medicament
    T88.8   Other specified complications of surgical and medical care, not elsewhere classified
    T88.9   Complication of surgical and medical care, unspecified

Chapter 20

External Causes of Morbidity

Chapter 20 of the ICD-10-CM Tabular List classifies external causes of morbidity. It includes categories V01 through Y98, which are arranged in the following blocks:

V00–X58   Accidents
    V00–V99   Transport accidents
        V00–V09   Pedestrian injured in transport accident
        V10–V19   Pedal cyclist injured in transport accident
        V20–V29   Motorcycle rider injured in transport accident
        V30–V39   Occupant of three-wheeled motor vehicle injured in transport accident
        V40–V49   Car occupant injured in transport accident
        V50–V59   Occupant of pick-up truck or van injured in transport accident
        V60–V69   Occupant of heavy transport vehicle injured in transport accident
        V70–V79   Bus occupant injured in transport accident
        V80–V89   Other land transport accidents
        V90–V94   Water transport accidents
        V95–V97   Air and space transport accidents
        V98–V99   Other and unspecified transport accidents
    W00–X58   Other external causes of accidental injury
        W00–W19   Falls
        W20–W49   Exposure to inanimate mechanical forces
        W50–W64   Exposure to animate mechanical forces
        W65–W74   Accidental drowning and submersion
        W85–W99   Exposure to electric current, radiation and extreme ambient air temperature and pressure
        X00–X09   Exposure to smoke, fire and flames
        X10–X19   Contact with heat and hot substances
        X30–X39   Exposure to forces of nature
        X52, X58   Accidental exposure to other specified factors
X71–X83   Intentional self-harm
X92–Y08   Assault
Y21–Y33   Event of undetermined intent
Y35–Y38   Legal intervention, operations of war, military operations, and terrorism

Y62–Y84 Complications of medical and surgical care

    Y62–Y69 Misadventures to patients during surgical and medical care

    Y70–Y82 Medical devices associated with adverse incidents in diagnostic and therapeutic use

    Y83–Y84 Surgical and other medical procedures as the cause of abnormal reaction of the patient, or of later complication, without mention of misadventure at the time of the procedure

Y90–Y98 Supplementary factors related to causes of morbidity classified elsewhere

Title Changes

A number of block, category, and subcategory title changes have been made in chapter 20 of ICD-10-CM. A few examples of these changes include the following:

ICD-9-CM: Accidental Falls (E880–E888)
ICD-10-CM: Falls (W00–W19)

ICD-9-CM: E884.0   Fall from playground equipment
ICD-10-CM: W09   Fall on and from playground equipment

ICD-9-CM: E883.0   Accident from diving or jumping into water [swimming pool]
ICD-10-CM: W16   Fall, jump or diving into water

Additions, Deletions, and Combinations

When chapter 20 is compared with the E codes in the Supplementary Classification of External Causes of Injury and Poisoning in ICD-9-CM, it is evident that many codes have been added, deleted, combined, or moved to another section or chapter. Examples of codes moved from section to another include the following:

- In ICD-9-CM, the E codes (Supplementary Classification of External Causes of Injury and Poisoning) are located at the end of the Tabular List; in ICD-10-CM, these codes follow chapter 19, Injury, poisoning and certain other consequences of external causes.

- In ICD-9-CM, the late effect codes for external causes are located in various subchapters of the Supplementary Classification; in ICD-10-CM, all late effects can be noted by the addition of the sequela extension (q) to the code for each intent (accidents, suicide, falls, and so on).

ICD-9-CM codes E850 through E858, Accidental Poisoning by Drugs, Medicinal Substances, and Biological Substances, and E860 through E869, Accidental Poisonings by Other Solid and Liquid Substances, Gases, and Vapors, have been moved in ICD-10-CM. For example, codes from the T36 through T50 category range identify the specific substances for poisoning by, adverse effects of, and underdosing of drugs, medicaments, and biological substances. In addition, codes from the T51 through T65 category range identify the toxic effects of nonmedicinal substances and identify the poisoning as accidental or unintentional. For example:

ICD-9-CM: E856   Accidental poisoning by antibiotics
               E860.4   Fusel oil
ICD-10-CM: T36.0x1   Poisoning by penicillins, accidental (unintentional)
               T51.3x1   Toxic effect of fusel oil, accidental (unintentional)

A specific code for exposure to radon, X39.01, has been added to ICD-10-CM.

Expansions

A number of codes for external causes of morbidity have been expanded in ICD-10-CM.

Subcategory Codes Given a Category Code

In numerous instances, conditions included as subcategory codes in ICD-9-CM have been given a specific category code in ICD-10-CM, which expands the codes at the fourth-, fifth-, or sixth-character level. In addition, in many instances in ICD-10-CM, extensions can be added to each of the codes from the category to indicate initial encounter, subsequent encounter, or sequelae. For example:

ICD-9-CM: E884.0   Fall from playground equipment
ICD-10-CM: W09   Fall on and from playground equipment
The following 7th character extensions are to be added to each code from category W09:
    a   initial encounter
    d   subsequent encounter
    q   sequelae
W09.0   Fall on or from playground slide
W09.1   Fall from playground swing
W09.2   Fall on or from jungle gym
W09.8   Fall on or from other playground equipment

ICD-9-CM: E883.0   Accident from diving or jumping into water [swimming pool]
ICD-10-CM: W16   Fall, jump or diving into water
The following 7th character extensions are to be added to each code from category W16:
    a   initial encounter
    d   subsequent encounter
    q   sequelae
W16.0   Fall into swimming pool
    W16.01   Fall into swimming pool striking water surface
        W16.011   Fall into swimming pool striking water surface causing drowning and submersion
        W16.012   Fall into swimming pool striking water surface causing other injury
    W16.02   Fall into swimming pool striking bottom
        W16.021   Fall into swimming pool striking bottom causing drowning and submersion
        W16.022   Fall into swimming pool striking bottom causing other injury
    W16.03   Fall into swimming pool striking wall
        W16.031   Fall into swimming pool striking wall causing drowning and submersion
        W16.032   Fall into swimming pool striking wall causing other injury
W16.1   Fall into natural body of water
    W16.11   Fall into natural body of water striking water surface
        W16.111   Fall into natural body of water striking water surface causing drowning and submersion
        W16.112   Fall into natural body of water striking water surface causing other injury

W16.12 Fall into natural body of water striking bottom
　　　　W16.121 Fall into natural body of water striking bottom causing drowning and submersion
　　　　W16.122 Fall into natural body of water striking bottom causing other injury
W16.13 Fall into natural body of water striking side
　　　　W16.131 Fall into natural body of water striking side causing drowning and submersion
　　　　W16.132 Fall into natural body of water striking side causing other injury
W16.2 Fall in (into) filled bathtub or bucket of water
　W16.21 Fall in (into) filled bathtub
　　　　W16.211 Fall in (into) filled bathtub causing drowning and submersion
　　　　W16.212 Fall in (into) filled bathtub causing other injury
　W16.22 Fall in (into) bucket of water
　　　　W16.221 Fall in (into) bucket of water causing drowning and submersion
　　　　W16.222 Fall in (into) bucket of water causing other injury
W16.3 Fall into other water
　W16.31 Fall into other water striking water surface
　　　　W16.311 Fall into other water striking water surface causing drowning and submersion
　　　　W16.312 Fall into other water striking water surface causing other injury
　W16.32 Fall into other water striking bottom
　　　　W16.321 Fall into other water striking bottom causing drowning and submersion
　　　　W16.322 Fall into other water striking bottom causing other injury
　W16.33 Fall into other water striking wall
　　　　W16.331 Fall into other water striking wall causing drowning and submersion
　　　　W16.332 Fall into other water striking wall causing other injury
W16.4 Fall into unspecified water
　W16.41 Fall into unspecified water causing drowning and submersion
　W16.42 Fall into unspecified water causing other injury
W16.5 Jumping or diving into swimming pool
　W16.51 Jumping or diving into swimming pool striking water surface
　　　　W16.511 Jumping or diving into swimming pool striking water surface causing drowning and submersion
　　　　W16.512 Jumping or diving into swimming pool striking water surface causing other injury

W16.52   Jumping or diving into swimming pool striking bottom

      W16.521   Jumping or diving into swimming pool striking bottom causing drowning and submersion

      W16.522   Jumping or diving into swimming pool striking bottom causing other injury

W16.53   Jumping or diving into swimming pool striking wall

      W16.531   Jumping or diving into swimming pool striking wall causing drowning and submersion

      W16.532   Jumping or diving into swimming pool striking wall causing other injury

W16.6   Jumping or diving into natural body of water

   W16.61   Jumping or diving into natural body of water striking water surface

      W16.611   Jumping or diving into natural body of water striking water surface causing drowning and submersion

      W16.612   Jumping or diving into natural body of water striking water surface causing other injury

   W16.62   Jumping or diving into natural body of water striking bottom

      W16.621   Jumping or diving into natural body of water striking bottom causing drowning and submersion

      W16.622   Jumping or diving into natural body of water striking bottom causing other injury

W16.7   Jumping or diving from boat

   W16.71   Jumping or diving from boat striking water surface

      W16.711   Jumping or diving from boat striking water surface causing drowning and submersion

      W16.712   Jumping or diving from boat striking water surface causing other injury

   W16.72   Jumping or diving from boat striking bottom

      W16.721   Jumping or diving from boat striking bottom causing drowning and submersion

      W16.722   Jumping or diving from boat striking bottom causing other injury

W16.8   Jumping or diving into other water

   W16.81   Jumping or diving into other water striking water surface

      W16.811   Jumping or diving into other water striking water surface causing drowning and submersion

      W16.812   Jumping or diving into other water striking water surface causing other injury

	W16.82	Jumping or diving into other water striking bottom
		W16.821 Jumping or diving into other water striking bottom causing drowning and submersion
		W16.822 Jumping or diving into other water striking bottom causing other injury
	W16.83	Jumping or diving into other water striking wall
		W16.831 Jumping or diving into other water striking wall causing drowning and submersion
		W16.832 Jumping or diving into other water striking wall causing other injury
W16.9		Jumping or diving into unspecified water
	W16.91	Jumping or diving into unspecified water causing drowning and submersion
	W16.92	Jumping or diving into unspecified water causing other injury

Transport Accidents

In ICD-9-CM, under the sections for transport accidents, the category codes identify the specific type of transport accidents and the fourth digits identify the injured individual. For example:

E819   Motor vehicle traffic accident of unspecified nature
The following fourth-digit subdivisions are for use with categories E810–E819 to identify the injured person:
.0   Driver of motor vehicle other than motorcycle
.1   Passenger in motor vehicle other than motorcycle
.2   Motorcyclist
.3   Passenger on motorcycle
.4   Occupant of streetcar
.5   Rider of animal; occupant of animal-drawn vehicle
.6   Pedal cyclist
.7   Pedestrian
.8   Other specified person
.9   Unspecified person

In ICD-10-CM, however, the main axis for transport accidents is the injured individual's mode of transportation. Each section has been greatly expanded to include fourth, fifth, and even sixth characters. Code extensions in these sections also further explain types of encounters or sequelae.

Complications of Medical and Surgical Care

Complications of medical and surgical care have been greatly expanded in ICD-10-CM, and several new categories have been added. For example:

Complications of medical and surgical care (Y62–Y84)

Misadventures to patients during surgical and medical care (Y62–Y69)
Y62   Failure of sterile precautions during surgical and medical care
Y63   Failure in dosage during surgical and medical care
Y64   Contaminated medical or biological substances
Y65   Other misadventures during surgical and medical care

Medical devices associated with adverse incidents in diagnostic and therapeutic use (Y70–Y82)

Y70   Anesthesiology devices associated with adverse incidents
Y71   Cardiovascular devices associated with adverse incidents
Y72   Otorhinolaryngological devices associated with adverse incidents
Y73   Gastroenterology and urology devices associated with adverse incidents
Y74   General hospital and personal-use devices associated with adverse incidents
Y75   Neurological devices associated with adverse incidents associated with adverse incidents
Y76   Obstetric and gynecological devices associated with adverse incidents
Y77   Ophthalmic devices associated with adverse incidents
Y78   Radiological devices associated with adverse incidents
Y79   Orthopedic devices associated with adverse incidents
Y80   Physical medicine devices associated with adverse incidents
Y81   General- and plastic-surgery devices associated with adverse incidents
Y82   Other and unspecified medical devices associated with adverse incidents

Surgical and other medical procedures as the cause of abnormal reaction of the patient, or of later complication, without mention of misadventure at the time of the procedure (Y83–Y84)

Y83   Surgical operation and other surgical procedures as the cause of abnormal reaction of the patient, or of later complication, without mention of misadventure at the time of the procedure
Y84   Other medical procedures as the cause of abnormal reaction of the patient, or of later complication, without mention of misadventure at the time of the procedure

Four-character codes under all of the preceding categories provide greater specificity.

Place of Occurrence

Category E849, Place of occurrence, in ICD-9-CM has been greatly expanded in category Y92 of ICD-10-CM to include fifth and sixth characters to further identify the specific area of each place of occurrence (kitchen, dining room, bathroom, driveway, garage, swimming pool, garden or yard, and so on).

Activity Codes

ICD-10-CM category Y93 provides secondary codes to be used with other external cause codes to identify the patient's activity at the time the injury occurred. Activity codes should be assigned only to initial encounters for treatment, and only one code should be assigned to each case. Activity codes are assigned along with codes from category Y92 for the place of the accident's occurrence. Activity code Y93.9 should be assigned when there is no information on the patient's activity and when assigning a code would not be appropriate. Category Y93 requires the use of a seventh-character extension: numeral one for activities not related to work, numeral two for activities related to work, numeral three for activities related to student education, and numeral four for activities related to military service.

Chapter 21

Factors Influencing Health Status and Contact with Health Services

Chapter 21 of the ICD-10-CM Tabular List classifies the various factors that influence a patient's health status and contact with health services. The chapter includes categories Z00 through Z99, which are arranged in the following blocks:

Z00–Z13   Persons encountering health services for examination and investigation

Z14–Z15   Genetic carrier and genetic susceptibility to disease

Z16   Infection with drug-resistant microorganisms

Z20–Z28   Persons with potential health hazards related to communicable diseases

Z30–Z39   Persons encountering health services in circumstances related to reproduction

Z40–Z53   Persons encountering health services for specific procedures and health care

Z55–Z65   Persons with potential health hazards related to socioeconomic and psycho-social circumstances

Z66   Do not resuscitate [DNR] status

Z67   Blood type

Z69–Z76   Persons encountering health services in other circumstances

Z79–Z99   Persons with potential health hazards related to family and personal history and certain conditions influencing health status

Z codes represent the reason for encounter, but a corresponding procedure code must be used to identify the specific procedure performed.

Categories Z00 through Z99 are provided for occasions when circumstances other than a disease, an injury, or an external cause classifiable to categories A00 through Y89 is recorded as the reason for encounter. This situation arises in two ways:

1. When a person who may or may not be sick receives health services for a specific purpose, such as to receive limited medical care or services for a current condition, to donate an organ or tissue, to receive a prophylactic vaccination, or to discuss a problem that is in itself not a disease or injury

2. When some circumstance or problem is present that influences the person's health status but is not in itself a current illness or injury

Additions, Deletions, and Combinations

When ICD-10-CM chapter 21 is compared with ICD-9-CM V codes from the Supplementary Classification of Factors Influencing Health Status and Contact with Health Services (V01–V82), it is evident that some codes have been added, deleted, combined, or moved from one section or chapter to another. For example, code Z02.81, Encounter for paternity testing, and code Z66, Do not resuscitate, represent specific codes that have been added to the revised classification.

ICD-9-CM does not provide specific codes for bloodtypes. ICD-10-CM category Z67, Bloodtype, in contrast, does provide specific codes for bloodtypes, as follows:

Z67 Bloodtype
    Z67.1 Type A blood
        Z67.10 Type A blood, Rh positive
        Z67.11 Type A blood, Rh negative
    Z67.2 Type B blood
        Z67.20 Type B blood, Rh positive
        Z67.21 Type B blood, Rh negative
    Z67.3 Type AB blood
        Z67.30 Type AB blood, Rh positive
        Z67.31 Type AB blood, Rh negative
    Z67.4 Type O blood
        Z67.40 Type O blood, Rh positive
        Z67.41 Type O blood, Rh negative
    Z67.9 Unspecified blood type
        Z67.90 Unspecified bloodtype, Rh positive
        Z67.91 Unspecified bloodtype, Rh negative

In some rare instances, ICD-10-CM is less specific than ICD-9-CM. One example is ICD-10-CM category Z16, Infection with drug-resistant microorganisms. This category is similar to ICD-9-CM category V09, Infection with drug-resistant microorganism. However, category V09 has several fourth- and fifth-digit codes that report the specific drugs to which the organism is resistant. The corresponding ICD-10-CM category (Z16) includes no further breakdown, but users are instructed to code first the infection.

Another example of decreased specificity in ICD-10-CM is code Z23, Encounter for immunization. This code is not broken down any further. In ICD-9-CM, category codes V03, V04, V05, and V06 are used to identify the type of immunization.

No major changes have been made in ICD-10-CM categories Z30 through Z39, Persons encountering health services in circumstances related to reproduction, with the exception of code Z33.2, Encounter for elective termination of pregnancy. As noted earlier, codes for elective abortion in ICD-9-CM are in the chapter on pregnancy, delivery, and puerperium. In ICD-10-CM the category for elective abortion is in chapter 21. This category excludes, of course, spontaneous abortion.

ICD-10-CM category Z36, Encounter for antenatal screening, does not include fourth-, fifth-, or sixth-character subclassifications. In ICD-9-CM, however, category V28, Antenatal screening, provides further specificity about the purpose of the screening.

Expansions

A number of codes for factors that influence health status and contact with health services have been expanded in ICD-10-CM.

Increased Specificity for Codes Related to Different Types of Examinations

Most of the codes within Z00 through Z13, Persons encountering health services for examinations, are very similar to ones found in ICD-9-CM, but with increased specificity. For example:

ICD-9-CM: V70.0   Routine general medical examination at a health care facility
ICD-10-CM: Z00.01 Encounter for general medical examination
        General physical examination, routine blood work and any associated radiology examinations

        Excludes 1:   routine laboratory examination without physical examination (Z00.02–)
                routine radiology examination without physical examination (Z00.03–)

        Z00.010 Encounter for general medical examination without abnormal findings
        Z00.011 Encounter for general medical examination with abnormal findings
                Use additional code to identify abnormal findings

ICD-9-CM: V72.5   Radiological examination not elsewhere classified
ICD-10-CM: Z00.03 Encounter for general radiology examination
        Encounter for routine chest X-ray

        Excludes 1:   encounter for general medical examination with radiology examination (Z00.01–)
                encounter for radiology examination for diagnostic purposes—code to signs and symptoms

        Z00.030 Encounter for general radiology examination without abnormal finding
        Z00.031 Encounter for general radiology examination with abnormal findings
                Use additional code to identify abnormal findings

Note that users are instructed to identify the results of the examination when abnormal findings are found. This instruction is a departure from the ICD-9-CM coding guidelines on the use of codes for routine examinations.

ICD-10-CM code Z01.3 is used for a routine encounter for examination of blood pressure. Fifth characters indicate the presence or absence of abnormal findings. Again, any abnormal results should be reported.

ICD-10-CM provides greater specificity for codes related to other types of examinations. For example:

ICD-9-CM: V70.3   Other medical examination for administrative purposes
               V70.4   Examination for medicolegal reasons
               V70.5   Health examination of defined subpopulations
ICD-10-CM: Z02   Encounter for administrative examination
        Z02.0   Encounter for examination for admission to educational institution
        Z02.1   Encounter for pre-employment examination
        Z02.2   Encounter for examination for admission to residential institution
        Z02.3   Encounter for examination for recruitment to armed forces
        Z02.4   Encounter for examination for driving license

Z02.5   Encounter for examination for participation in sports
Z02.6   Encounter for examination for insurance purposes
Z02.7   Encounter for issue of medical certificate
  Z02.71   Encounter for disability determination
  Z02.79   Encounter for issue of other medical certificate
Z02.8   Encounter for other administrative examinations
  Z02.81   Encounter for paternity testing
  Z02.82   Encounter for adoption services
  Z02.83   Encounter for blood-alcohol and blood-drug test
  Z02.89   Encounter for other administrative examinations
Z02.9   Encounter for administrative examinations, unspecified

In ICD-CM-10, category codes Z08 and Z09 are used to report encounters for follow-up examination after completed treatment for malignant neoplasms (Z08) and for conditions other than malignant neoplasms (Z09). In ICD-9-CM, these types of follow-up encounters are reported using codes from category V67.

ICD-10-CM categories Z11 through Z13 are used to report encounters for specific screening examinations. Screening is described as testing for disease or disease precursors in asymptomatic individuals so that early detection and treatment can be provided for those who test positive for the disease. Excludes statements under each of these categories instruct users to code to signs or symptoms when screening tests are performed as part of a diagnostic workup.

Immunization Not Carried Out

ICD-10-CM category code Z28, Immunization not carried out, has fourth and fifth characters that identify the specific reason the immunization was not carried out.

Z28.0   Immunization not carried out because of contraindication
 Z28.1   Immunization not carried out because of patient's decision for reasons of belief or group pressure
 Z28.2   Immunization not carried out because of patient's decision for other and unspecified reason
  Z28.20   Immunization not carried out because of patient's decision for unspecified reason
  Z28.29   Immunization not carried out because of patient's decision for other reason
 Z28.8   Immunization not carried out for other reason
  Z28.81   Immunization not carried out due to patient's having had the disease
  Z28.89   Immunization not carried out for other reason
 Z28.9   Immunization not carried out for unspecified reason

Expansions for Specific Procedures

The codes in categories Z40 through Z53, Persons encountering health services for specific procedures and health care, are intended for use to indicate a reason for care. They may be used for patients who already have been treated for a disease or injury but who are receiving after-care or prophylactic care, convalescent care, or care to consolidate the treatment or to deal with residual states. The majority of the code descriptions are very similar to ICD-9-CM, but ICD-10-CM provides codes to identify laterality in some instances. For example:

ICD-9-CM: V52.0   Fitting and adjustment of artificial arm (complete) (partial)
ICD-10-CM: Z44.0   Encounter for fitting and adjustment of artificial arm
　　　　　　　 Z44.00   Encounter for fitting and adjustment of unspecified artificial
　　　　　　　　　　　 arm
　　　　　　　　　　　 Z44.001   Encounter for fitting and adjustment of unspecified
　　　　　　　　　　　　　　　　 right artificial arm
　　　　　　　　　　　 Z44.002   Encounter for fitting and adjustment of unspecified
　　　　　　　　　　　　　　　　 left artificial arm
　　　　　　　　　　　 Z44.009   Encounter for fitting and adjustment of unspecified
　　　　　　　　　　　　　　　　 artificial arm, unspecified arm
　　　　　　　 Z44.01   Encounter for fitting and adjustment of complete artificial
　　　　　　　　　　　 arm
　　　　　　　　　　　 Z44.011   Encounter for fitting and adjustment of complete
　　　　　　　　　　　　　　　　 right artificial arm
　　　　　　　　　　　 Z44.012   Encounter for fitting and adjustment of complete
　　　　　　　　　　　　　　　　 left artificial arm
　　　　　　　　　　　 Z44.019   Encounter for fitting and adjustment of complete
　　　　　　　　　　　　　　　　 artificial arm, unspecified arm

Increased Specificity for Health Hazards Related to Socioeconomic and Psychosocial Circumstances

In ICD-10-CM categories Z55 through Z65, Persons with potential health hazards related to socioeconomic and psychosocial circumstances, codes provide a high level of specificity. For example:

ICD-9-CM: V62.3   Educational circumstances
ICD-10-CM: Z55   Problems related to education and literacy
　　　　　　　 Z55.0   Illiteracy and low-level literacy
　　　　　　　 Z55.1   Schooling unavailable and unattainable
　　　　　　　 Z55.2   Failed school examinations
　　　　　　　 Z55.3   Underachievement in school
　　　　　　　 Z55.4   Educational maladjustment and discord with teachers and
　　　　　　　　　　　 classmates
　　　　　　　 Z55.8   Other problems related to education and literacy
　　　　　　　 Z55.9   Problems related to education and literacy, unspecified

ICD-9-CM: V62.0   Unemployment
ICD-10-CM: Z56   Problems related to employment and unemployment
　　　　　　　 Z56.0   Unemployment, unspecified
　　　　　　　 Z56.1   Change of job
　　　　　　　 Z56.2   Threat of job loss
　　　　　　　 Z56.3   Stressful work schedule
　　　　　　　 Z56.4   Discord with boss and workmates
　　　　　　　 Z56.5   Uncongenial work environment
　　　　　　　 Z56.6   Other physical and mental strain related to work
　　　　　　　 Z56.8   Other problems related to employment
　　　　　　　　　　　 Z56.81   Sexual harassment on the job
　　　　　　　　　　　 Z56.89   Other problems related to employment
　　　　　　　 Z56.9   Unspecified problems related to employment

ICD-9-CM: V62.1   Adverse effects of work environment

ICD-10-CM: Z57   Occupational exposure to risk factors

    Z57.0   Occupational exposure to noise

    Z57.1   Occupational exposure to radiation

    Z57.2   Occupational exposure to dust

    Z57.3   Occupational exposure to the air contaminants

        Z57.31   Occupational exposure to environmental tobacco smoke

        Z57.39   Occupational exposure to other air contaminants

    Z57.4   Occupational exposure to toxic agents in agriculture

    Z57.5   Occupational exposure to toxic agents in other industries

    Z57.6   Occupational exposure to extreme temperature

    Z57.7   Occupational exposure to vibration

    Z57.8   Occupational exposure to risk factors

    Z57.9   Occupational exposure to unspecified risk factor

Z58   Problems related to physical environment

    Z58.0   Exposure to noise

    Z58.1   Exposure to air pollution

    Z58.2   Exposure to water pollution

    Z58.3   Exposure to oil pollution

    Z58.4   Exposure to radiation

    Z58.5   Exposure to other pollution

    Z58.6   Inadequate drinking-water supply

    Z58.8   Other problems related to physical environment

        Z58.81   Problems related to exposure to lead

        Z58.82   Problems related to exposure to asbestos

        Z58.89   Other problems related to physical environment

    Z58.9   Problems related to physical environment, unspecified

Other interesting ICD-10-CM chapter 21 category codes include:

Z62   Other problems related to upbringing

    Z62.0   Inadequate parental supervision and control

    Z62.1   Parental overprotection

    Z62.2   Institutional upbringing

    Z62.3   Hostility toward and scapegoating of child

    Z62.6   Inappropriate parental pressure and other abnormal qualities of upbringing

        Z62.8   Other specified problems related to upbringing

        Z62.9   Problem related to upbringing, unspecified

Z65   Problems related to other psychosocial circumstances

    Z65.0   Conviction in civil and criminal proceedings without imprisonment

    Z65.1   Imprisonment and other incarceration

    Z65.2   Problems related to release from prison

    Z65.3   Problems related to other legal circumstances

    Z65.4   Victim of crime and terrorism

    Z65.5   Exposure to disaster, war and other hostilities

    Z65.8   Other specified problems related to psychosocial circumstances

    Z65.9   Problem related to unspecified psychosocial circumstances

Increased Specificity for Codes Used to Report Counseling

ICD-10-CM provides specificity for the codes in categories Z69 through Z76, Persons encountering health services in other circumstances, that are used to report counseling. For example, sexual counseling is assigned to code V65.49, Other specified counseling, in ICD-9-CM. The codes in ICD-10-CM include the following:

Z70   Counseling related to sexual attitude, behavior and orientation
    Z70.0   Counseling related to sexual attitude
    Z70.1   Counseling related to patient's sexual behavior and orientation
    Z70.2   Counseling related to sexual behavior and orientation of third party
    Z70.3   Counseling related to combined concerns regarding sexual attitude, behavior and orientation
    Z70.8   Other sexual counseling
    Z70.9   Sex counseling, unspecified

Increased Specificity to Report Personal and Family History of Various Conditions

In ICD-10-CM, codes from categories Z79 through Z99, Persons with potential health hazards related to family and personal history and certain conditions influencing health status, are used to report both personal and family history of various conditions. When coding personal history of malignant neoplasms, it is possible to code both a personal history of a primary malignant neoplasm and a secondary malignant neoplasm, which was not possible in ICD-9-CM.

In addition, ICD-10-CM provides category Z79 to identify long-term (current) drug therapy with fourth characters identifying the type of drugs. Users of ICD-10-CM are reminded to code also any encounter for therapeutic drug-level monitoring (Z51.81). The *excludes* statement reminds users that drug abuse and dependence are not classified to category Z79 but, rather, to categories F11 through F19. Examples of codes in Z79, Long-term (current) drug therapy, include:

Z79.0   Long-term (current) uses of anticoagulants
Z79.1   Long-term (current) uses of antithrombotics/antiplatelets
Z79.2   Long-term (current) use of anti-inflammatories

There also are codes to identify the status of allergies to drugs, medicaments, and biological substances as well as to foods, insects, and nonmedicinal substances such as latex. Some examples include:

Z88.0   Allergy status to penicillin
Z88.1   Allergy status to other antibiotic agents
Z88.2   Allergy status to sulfonamides

Z91.01   Food allergy status
    Z91.010   Allergy to peanuts
    Z91.011   Allergy to milk products
    Z91.012   Allergy to eggs
    Z91.013   Allergy to seafood
    Z91.018   Allergy to other foods

Z91.0   Allergy status, other than to drugs and biological substances
    Z91.04   Nonmedicinal substance allergy status
        Z91.040   Latex allergy status

Some of the other codes in this block are used to report conditions such as:

- Artificial opening status

- Transplanted organ or tissue status

- Presence of cardiac and vascular implants and grafts

- Presence of other functional implants

- Presence of devices

- Postsurgical states and dependence on enabling machines and devices (respirators, ventilators, and so on)

ICD-10-CM categories Z79 through Z99 include a number of interesting codes. Just a few examples include:

Z91.3	Unhealthy sleep–wake schedule
Z91.5	Personal history of self-harm
Z91.71	Low birth weight status
Z92.3	Personal history of irradiation
Z96.1	Presence of intraocular lens
Z96.3	Presence of artificial larynx
Z98.3	Post therapeutic collapse of lung status
Z98.51	Tubal ligation status
Z98.52	Vasectomy status
Z99.1	Dependence on respiratory/ventilator

Note that sixth characters identify the birth weight under code Z91.71.

Appendix

ICD-10-CM Coding Guidelines

Draft ICD-10-CM Official Guidelines
For Coding and Reporting for Acute Short-term and Long-term Hospital Inpatient and Physician Office and other Outpatient Encounters

Introduction

The National Center for Health Statistics (NCHS), one of the Centers for Disease Control and Prevention (CDC), an agency within the United States Department of Health and Human Services (DHHS), presents the following guidelines for coding and reporting using the International Classification of Diseases, 10th Revision, Clinical Modification (ICD-10-CM). These guidelines should be used as a companion document to the official government version of the ICD-10-CM.

The ICD-10-CM is a morbidity classification published by the United States for classifying diagnoses and reason for visits in all health care settings. The ICD-10-CM is based on the ICD-10, the statistical classification of disease published by the World Health Organization (WHO). The ICD-10 is used in the United States solely as a mortality classification for the coding of death certificates. A morbidity classification contains substantially more detail than is required in a mortality classification. It does include conditions that are potentially fatal, but which are, at least to some degree, treatable. No strictly fatal conditions, such as decapitation, are included, the exceptions being codes for stillbirth, and death NOS, for a patient who has died and is brought to an emergency department (ED) to be pronounced dead.

The United States is bound by international treaty to report mortality data to the WHO using ICD-10 codes. Where a note in the ICD-10-CM Tabular List indicates that a category or categories have been deactivated, it is a category from the ICD-10 that is not for use with the ICD-10-CM. The notes are for those who wish to compare data between ICD-10 and ICD-10-CM.

The ICD-10-CM is in the public domain, however, neither categories nor code titles may be altered in any way, except through the Coordination and Maintenance process, the annual updating procedure overseen jointly by NCHS and the Centers for Medicare and Medicaid Services (CMS).

There are no codes for procedures in the ICD-10-CM. Procedures are coded using the procedure classification appropriate for the encounter setting.

These guidelines for coding and reporting appear on the official government version of the ICD-10-CM and on the NCHS website. (add website address)

These conventions and guidelines apply to the proper use of ICD-10-CM for acute short-term and long-term hospital inpatient and physician office and other outpatient settings. The guidelines will be reviewed on an annual basis corresponding to the annual update to the ICD-10-CM. New guidelines will be written to correspond to new codes that are added to ICD-10-CM or for types of encounters for which no guidelines exist. The term "encounter" in these guidelines is used generally to mean a health care encounter, including an inpatient admission.

The guidelines are organized into several sections: Section 1, ICD-10-CM conventions, Section 2, General coding guidelines, and Section 3, Chapter-specific guidelines. The chapter-specific guidelines are sequenced in the same order they appear in the Tabular List. **It is necessary to review all sections of the guidelines to fully understand all of the rules and instructions needed to code properly.**

Table of Contents

Section I   ICD-10-CM Conventions
I.a   Format
I.b   Punctuation
I.c   Use of "and"
I.d   "Other specified" codes (NEC)
I.e   "Unspecified" codes (NOS)
I.f   Includes notes
I.g   Inclusion terms
I.h   Excludes notes
I.i   Code first/use additional code notes (etiology/manifestation paired codes)
I.j   Code also note
I.k   With/without note

Section II   General Coding Guidelines
II.a   Locating a code in the ICD-10-CM
II.b   Use of symptom codes with confirmed diagnoses
II.c   Acute and chronic conditions
II.d   Combination codes
II.e   Laterality
II.f   Selection of principal or first listed diagnosis
        II.f.1   Use of symptom codes as principal/first listed diagnosis
        II.f.2   Acute manifestation versus underlying condition
        II.f.3   Two or more diagnoses that equally meet the definition of principal diagnosis
        II.f.4   Original treatment plan not carried out
        II.f.5   Complications of surgery and other medical care
II.g   Selection of secondary diagnoses
        II.g.1   Previous conditions
        II.g.2   Abnormal test findings

Section III: Chapter-specific Guidelines
Chapter 1: Certain infectious and parasitic diseases
1.1 Human immunodeficiency virus [HIV] disease
        1.1.1   Sequencing of HIV codes
        1.1.2   HIV in a pregnant patient
        1.1.3   Encounter for testing for HIV
1.2 Sepsis
1.3 Infectious agents as the cause of diseases classified to other chapters
1.4 Nosocomial infections

Chapter 2: Neoplasms
2.1 Neoplasm Table
2.2 Use of pathology report
2.3 Morphology codes
2.4 Neoplasms of uncertain behavior versus neoplasms of unspecified behavior
2.5 Sequencing of neoplasm codes
2.6 Cancer in a pregnant patient
2.7 Malignant neoplasm without specific site
2.8 Encounters for chemotherapy and radiation therapy
2.9 Endocrine therapy

Chapter 3:   Diseases of the blood and blood-forming organs and certain disorders involving the immune mechanism
3.1 Intraoperative and postprocedural hematologic and immune system complications

Chapter 4: Endocrine, nutritional, and metabolic diseases
4.1 Diabetes mellitus
      4.1.1   Diabetes mellitus in a pregnant patient
      4.1.2   Diabetic patient who receives an organ(s) transplant
4.2 Intraoperative and postprocedural endocrine system complications

Chapter 5: Mental and behavioral disorders
5.1 ICD-10-CM and DSM-IV-TR
5.2 Alcohol and drug abuse and dependence
5.3 Dementia with behavioral disturbance

Chapter 6: Diseases of nervous system
6.1 Dominant/nondominant side
6.2 Parkinson's disease
6.3 Dementia
6.4 Intraoperative and postprocedural nervous system complications

Chapter 7: Diseases of the eye and adnexa
7.1 Laterality
7.2 Intraoperative and postprocedural ophthalmologic complications

Chapter 8: Diseases of the ear and mastoid process
8.1 Intraoperative and postprocedural auditory system complications

Chapter 9: Diseases of circulatory system
9.1 Rheumatic heart disease
9.2 Hypertension
      9.2.1   Hypertensive heart disease

9.2.2 Hypertensive renal disease

9.2.3 Hypertensive heart and renal disease

9.2.4 Hypertensive retinopathy

9.2.5 Secondary hypertension

9.2.6 Hypertension, controlled

9.2.7 Hypertension, uncontrolled

9.2.8 Elevated blood pressure

9.3 Atherosclerotic coronary artery disease and angina

9.4 Initial and subsequent acute myocardial infarction

9.5 Cardiac arrest

9.6 Cerebrovascular occlusion and stenosis and cerebral infarction

9.7 Stroke, not specified as hemorrhage or infarction

9.8 Sequelae of cerebrovascular disease

9.9 Intraoperative and postprocedural circulatory system complications

Chapter 10: Diseases of respiratory system

10.1 Chronic obstructive pulmonary disease (COPD)

10.2 Nosocomial respiratory infections

10.3 Intraoperative and postprocedural respiratory system complications

Chapter 11: Diseases of digestive system

11.1 Ulcers

11.2 Crohn's disease/Ulcerative colitis

11.3 Intraoperative and postprocedural digestive system complications

Chapter 12: Diseases of the skin and subcutaneous tissue

12.1 Dermatology codes and the use of an external cause

12.2 Decubitus ulcers and non-decubitus chronic ulcers of lower limb codes

12.3 Intraoperative and postprocedural dermatologic complications

Chapter 13: Diseases of the musculoskeletal system and connective tissue

13.1 Site and laterality

13.2 Acute/chronic/recurrent musculoskeletal conditions

13.3 Osteoporosis

13.4 Intraoperative and postprocedural musculoskeletal system complications

13.5 Pathologic fracture in neoplastic disease

Chapter 14: Diseases of the genitourinary system

14.1 Renal failure

14.2 Infertility

14.3 Hyperplasia of prostate

14.4 Hypertensive renal disease

14.5 Intraoperative and postprocedural genitourinary system complications

Chapter 15: Pregnancy, childbirth, and the puerperium

15.1   General Chapter 15 guidelines
15.2   Sequencing of obstetric (OB) codes
15.3   Trimesters
15.4   Complications of ectopic pregnancy, miscarriage, and other abnormal products of conception
15.5   Multiple gestations
15.6   HIV in a pregnant patient
15.7   Gestational diabetes
15.8   Pre-existing conditions versus conditions due to the pregnancy
15.9   Maternal care for fetal conditions
15.10   Fetal conditions
15.11   Outcome of delivery
15.12   Intrauterine death versus stillbirth
15.13   Encounter for full-term uncomplicated delivery
15.14   Encounter for cesarean delivery without indication
15.15   Routine prenatal visits
15.16   Encounter for termination of pregnancy
15.17   The postpartum period
15.18   Sequelae of complication of pregnancy, childbirth, and the puerperium
15.19   Encounter for contraceptive and procreative management
15.20   Encounter for antenatal screening

Chapter 16: Certain conditions originating in the newborn (perinatal) period

16.1   General Chapter 16 guidelines
16.2   Liveborn infant according to place of birth and type of delivery
16.3   Newborn (suspected to be) affected by maternal conditions
16.4   Congenital anomalies in a newborn
16.5   Prematurity and low birth weight
16.6   Low birth weight and immaturity status
16.7   Newborn affected by intrauterine procedure
16.8   Stillbirths

Chapter 17: Congenital malformations, deformations and chromosomal abnormalities

17.1   Coding of syndromes

Chapter 18: Symptoms, signs and abnormal clinical and laboratory findings, not elsewhere classified

18.1   General Chapter 18 guidelines
18.2   Severe sepsis and septic shock
18.3   Encounter for pain management
18.4   Falling
18.5   Glasgow coma scale
18.6   Death NOS

Chapter 19: Injury, poisoning and certain other consequences of external causes

19.1   Chapter 19 code extensions
    19.1.1 Extensions "a" and "d"
    19.1.2 Extension "q"
19.2   S codes
    19.2.1 Superficial and open wounds
    19.2.2 Fractures
        19.2.2.1   Fracture extensions
    19.2.3 Crush injuries
    19.2.4 Amputations
    19.2.5 Spinal cord injuries
    19.2.6 Use of an external cause code (chapter 20) with an injury code
19.3   T codes
    19.3.1 Burns and corrosions
        19.3.1.1   Non-healing or infected burns and corrosions
        19.3.1.2   Burn NOS, Corrosion NOS
        19.3.1.3   Burns and corrosions classified according to extent of body surface involved
        19.3.1.4   Use of an external cause code with burns and corrosions
        19.3.1.5   Sequelae of burns and corrosions
    19.3.2 Poisonings, toxic effects, adverse effects and underdosing
        19.3.2.1   5th character "x" place holder
        19.3.2.2   Sequencing of poisonings, toxic effects, adverse effects and underdosing
        19.3.2.3   Poisonings, toxic effects, adverse effects and underdosing in a pregnant patient
    19.3.3 Other T codes that include the external cause
    19.3.4 Adult and child abuse, neglect and other maltreatment
        19.3.4.1   Use of an external cause code with an abuse or neglect code
        19.3.4.2   Abuse and other maltreatment in a pregnant patient

19.3.5 Complications of surgical and medical care, not elsewhere classified
    19.3.5.1   Complication codes that include the external cause
    19.3.5.2   Mechanical complications
    19.3.5.3   Organ transplant complications
    19.3.5.4   Complications of care within the body system chapters

Chapter 20: External causes of morbidity
20.1   General Chapter 20 guidelines
20.2   External cause code extensions
20.3   Unintentional (accidental) injuries
    20.3.1 Transport accidents
    20.3.2 Falls
20.4   Assault
    20.4.1 Adult and child abuse, neglect and maltreatment
20.5   Undetermined intent
20.6   Legal interventions
20.7   Operations of war/military operations
20.8   Terrorism
20.9   Place of occurrence
20.10 Activity code

Chapter 21: Factors influencing health status and contact with health service
21.1   General Chapter 21 guidelines
21.2   The Z code categories
    21.2.1 General and administrative examinations
    21.2.2 Observation
    21.2.3 Follow-up
    21.2.4 Screening
    21.2.5 Contact/Exposure
    21.2.6 Status
    21.2.7 Encounter for immunization/Immunization not carried out
    21.2.8 Encounters for health services related to reproduction
    21.2.9 Aftercare
        21.2.9.1   Encounter for radiation therapy and chemotherapy
    21.2.10   Donor
    21.2.11   Counseling
    21.2.12   History (of)
    21.2.13   Miscellaneous Z codes
21.3   Z Code Table

Section I: ICD-10-CM Conventions

The conventions for the ICD-10-CM are the general rules for use of the classification independent of the guidelines. These conventions are incorporated within the Index and Tabular List of the ICD-10-CM as instructional notes. The conventions are applicable to all health care settings.

The conventions are as follows:

I.a Format
The ICD-10-CM is divided into the Index, an alphabetical list of terms and their corresponding code, and the Tabular List, a chronological list of codes divided into chapters based on body system or condition. The Index is divided into two parts, the Index to Diseases and Injury, and the Index to External Causes of Injury. Within the Index of Diseases and Injury there is a Neoplasm Table and a Table of Drugs and Chemicals. See guideline 2.1 for instructions on use of the Neoplasm Table and guideline 19.3.2 for instructions on the use of the Table of Drugs and Chemicals.

The ICD-10-CM uses an indented format for ease in reference. The Tabular List contains categories, subcategories and codes. Each character for all categories, subcategories and codes may be either a letter or a number. All categories are 3 characters. The first character of a category is a letter. The second and third characters are numbers. A 3 character category that has no further subdivision is equivalent to a code. Subcategories are either 4 or 5 characters. Subcategory characters may be either letters or numbers. Codes are either 4, 5 or 6 characters. That is, each level of subdivision after a category is a subcategory. The final level of subdivision is a code. The final character in a code may be either a letter or a number.

The ICD-10-CM utilizes dummy place holders, always the letter x. A dummy "x" is used as a 5th character place holder at certain 6 character codes to allow for future expansion. The best example of this is at the poisoning codes, categories T36-T50, and the toxic effect codes, categories T51-T65.

The 6th character for the codes at categories T36-T50 always indicates the intent:
unintentional (accidental)
intentional self-harm
assault
undetermined
or an adverse effect
or underdosing
The 6th character for the codes at categories T51-T65 always indicates the intent.

The 5th character x will permit the future expansion of these codes without disturbing the 6th character structure.

Certain categories have applicable 7th character extensions. The extension is required for all codes within the category, or as the notes in the tabular instruct. The extension must always be the 7th character in the data field. If a code is not a full 6 characters, a dummy place holder x must be used to fill in the empty characters when a 7th character extension is required.

All codes on the official version of the ICD-10-CM are in bold. **Only codes are permissible for reporting purposes, not categories or subcategories. For codes with applicable extensions the extension is required at the 7th character for reporting purposes.**

I.b Punctuation

[ ] Brackets are used in the Tabular List to enclose synonyms, alternative wording or explanatory phrases. Brackets are used in the Index to identify manifestation codes. (see-Code first/Use additional code convention)

( ) Parentheses are used in both the Index and Tabular List to enclose supplementary words which may be present or absent in the statement of a disease or procedure without affecting the code number to which it is assigned. The terms within the parentheses are referred to as nonessential modifiers.

: Colons are used in the Tabular List after an incomplete term which needs one or more of the modifiers following the colon to make it assignable to a given category.

I.c Use of "and"
When the term "and" is used in a narrative statement it represents and/or.

I.d "Other specified" codes (NEC)
Codes titled "Other..." or "Other specified..." in the Tabular List (usually a code with a 4th or 6th character 8 or z and fifth character 9) are for use when the information in the medical record provides detail for which a specific code does not exist.

The abbreviation NEC, "Not elsewhere classifiable" represents "other specified" in the ICD-10-CM. An index entry that states NEC directs the coder to an "other specified" code in the Tabular List (see- Inclusion terms).

I.e "Unspecified" codes (NOS)
Codes in the Tabular List with "Unspecified..." in the title (usually a code with a 4th or 6th character 9 and 5th character 0) are for use when the information in the medical record is insufficient to assign a more specific code. The abbreviation NOS, "Not otherwise specified", in the Tabular List is the equivalent of unspecified.

I.f Includes notes

The word "Includes" appears immediately under certain categories to further define, or give examples of, the content of the category.

I.g Inclusion terms

Lists of terms are included under some codes. These terms are some of the conditions for which that code number is to be used. The terms may be synonyms of the code title, or, in the case of "other specified" codes, the terms are a list of some of the various conditions assigned to that code. The inclusion terms are not necessarily exhaustive. Additional terms found only in the Index may also be assigned to a code.

I.h Excludes notes

The ICD-10-CM has two types of excludes notes. Each note has a different definition for use but they are all similar in that they indicate that codes excluded from each other are independent of each other.

Excludes1

A type 1 Excludes note is a pure excludes. It means "NOT CODED HERE!" An Excludes1 note indicates that the code excluded should never be used at the same time as the code above the Excludes1 note. An Excludes1 is for used for when two conditions cannot occur together, such as a congenital form versus an acquired form of the same condition.

Excludes2

A type 2 excludes note represents "Not included here". An excludes2 note indicates that the condition excluded is not part of the condition represented by the code, from but a patient may have both conditions at the same time. When an Excludes2 note appears under a code, it is acceptable to use both the code and the excluded code together.

I.i Code first/use additional code notes (etiology/manifestation paired codes)

Certain conditions have both an underlying etiology and multiple body system manifestations due to the underlying etiology. For such conditions the ICD-10-CM has a coding convention that requires the underlying condition be sequenced first followed by the manifestation. Wherever such a combination exists there is a "use additional code" note at the etiology code, and a "code first" note at the manifestation code. These instructional notes indicate the proper sequencing order of the codes, etiology followed by manifestation.

In most cases the manifestation codes will have in the code title, "in diseases classified elsewhere." Codes with this title are a component of the etiology/ manifestation convention. The code title indicates that it is a manifestation code. "In diseases classified elsewhere" codes are never permitted to be used as first listed or principal diagnosis codes. They must be used in conjunction with an underlying condition code and they must be listed following the underlying condition. See category F02 for an example of this convention.

In addition to the notes in the Tabular list, these conditions also have a specific index entry structure. In the Index both conditions are listed together with the etiology code first followed by the manifestation codes in brackets. The code in brackets is always to be sequenced second.

In some circumstances, more than two codes may be required to fully describe a condition. In these cases a "use additional code" note will be present at a complication or manifestation code to indicate that more codes are needed. The additional codes used are secondary codes that are to be sequenced following any underlying cause and following the main manifestation. See code R65.2 for an example of this convention.

I.j Code also note

A "code also" note instructs that two codes may be required to fully describe a condition, but the sequencing of the two codes depends on the severity of the conditions and the reason for the encounter. See subcategory H05.32 for an example of this convention.

I.k With/without note

When "with" and "without" are the two options for the final character of a set of codes, the default is always "without." For five-character codes, a "0" as the fifth-position character represents "without", and "1" represents "with." For six-character codes, the sixth-position character "1" represents "with" and "9" represents "without."

Section II: General Coding Guidelines

The listing of diagnoses in the medical record is the responsibility of the attending physician. A joint effort between the attending physician and the coder is essential to achieve complete and accurate documentation and code assignment. These guidelines have been developed to assist both the physician and the coder in identifying those diagnoses that are to be assigned.

II.a Locating a code in the ICD-10-CM

To select a code in the classification that corresponds to a diagnosis or reason for visit documented in a medical record, first locate the term in the Index, then verify the code in the Tabular List. Read and be guided by instructional notations that appear in both the Index and the Tabular List.

It is essential to use both the Index and Tabular List when locating and assigning a code. The index does not always provide the full code. Selection of the full code, including laterality and any applicable extensions can only be done in the Tabular list. A - dash at the end of an index entry indicates that additional characters are required. Even if a dash is not included at the index entry, it is necessary to refer to the Tabular list to verify that no extension is required.

II.b Use of symptom codes with confirmed diagnoses

A symptom code should not be used with a confirmed diagnosis if the symptom is integral to the diagnosis, such as the use of a chest pain code with an acute myocardial infarction (MI) code. Pain is integral to an acute MI.

A symptom code should be used with a confirmed diagnosis if the symptom is not always associated with that diagnosis, such as the use various signs and symptom associated with complex syndromes.

II.c Acute and chronic conditions

If the same condition is described as both acute (subacute) and chronic, and separate subentries exist in the Index at the same indentation level, code both and sequence the acute (subacute) code first.

II.d Combination codes

A combination code is a single code used to classify:
two diagnoses, or
A diagnosis with an associated sign or symptom, or
A diagnosis with an associated complication

Combination codes are identified by referring to subterm entries in the Index and by reading the Includes and Exclusion notes in the Tabular List.

Assign only the combination code when that code fully identifies the diagnostic conditions involved or when the Index so directs. Multiple codes should not be used when the classification provides a combination code that clearly identifies all of the elements documented in the diagnosis. When the combination code lacks the necessary specificity to fully describe all elements of a diagnosis, an additional code(s) may be used.

II.e Laterality

For bilateral sites, the final character of the codes in the ICD-10-CM indicate laterality. The right side is always character 1, the left side character 2. In those cases where a bilateral code is provided the bilateral character is always 3. An unspecified side code is also provided should the side not be identified in the medical record. The unspecified side is either a character 0 or 9 depending on whether it is a 5th or 6th character.

II.f Selection of principal or first listed diagnosis

The code sequenced first on a medical record at the end of an encounter is most important because it defines the main reason for the encounter as determined at the end of the encounter. In the inpatient setting, the first code listed on a medical record is referred to as the principal diagnosis. In all other health care settings it is referred to as the first listed code.

The principal diagnosis is defined in the Uniform Hospital Discharge Data Set (UHDDS) as "that condition established after study to be chiefly responsible for occasioning the admission of the patient to the hospital for care". These data elements and their definitions can be found in the July 31, 1985, Federal Register (Vol. 50, No, 147), pp. 31038-40. The UHDDS definition also applies in selection of the first listed diagnosis code in other health care settings.

Selection of principal diagnosis/first listed code is based first on the conventions in the classification that provide sequencing instructions. If no sequencing instructions apply then sequencing is based on the condition(s) that brought the patient into the hospital or physician office and which condition was the primary focus of treatment. Conditions present on admission that receive treatment, but that do not meet the definition of principal diagnosis, should be coded as additional codes.

Additional guidelines on the selection of the principal/first listed code are as follows:

II.f.1 Use of symptom codes as principal/first listed diagnosis

A sign or symptom code (generally codes from Chapter 18 but signs and symptoms codes can be found in the body system chapters as well) is not to be used as a principal diagnosis when a definitive diagnosis for the sign or symptom has been established.

A sign or symptom code is to be used as principal/first listed if no definitive diagnosis is established at the time of coding. If the diagnosis is confirmed (e.g., an X-ray confirms a fracture, a pathology or laboratory report confirms a diagnosis) prior to coding the encounter, the confirmed diagnosis code should be used.

II.f.2 Acute manifestation versus underlying condition

With the UHDDS definition of principal diagnosis in mind, it is generally an underlying condition that precipitates the need for an admission since treatment of the underlying condition generally resolves any associated acute manifestations and is the primary focus of treatment. If the acute manifestation is immediately life-threatening and primary treatment is directed at the acute manifestation the acute manifestation should be sequenced before the underlying condition. If the acute manifestation is not the primary focus of treatment the underlying condition should be sequenced first.

This guideline is also based on the fact that the classification has the etiology/manifestation convention that requires that the underlying etiology take sequencing precedence over the acute manifestation.

There are many combination codes that include both the etiology and an acute manifestation, in which case the single combination code is assigned as the principal/first listed diagnosis and no sequencing decision is necessary.

Sequencing examples of acute manifestation versus underlying condition can be found in the chapter specific guidelines.

II.f.3 Two or more diagnoses that equally meet the definition of principal diagnosis/first listed

In the instance when two or more confirmed diagnoses equally meet the criteria for principal/first listed diagnosis as determined by the circumstances of admission, diagnostic workup and/or therapy provided, and the Index, Tabular List and coding guidelines do not provide sequencing direction, any one of the diagnoses may be sequenced first. This rule also applies to the outpatient setting.

II.f.4 Original treatment plan not carried out

If anticipated treatment is not carried out due to unforeseen circumstances, the principal diagnosis/first listed code remains the condition or diagnosis that was planned to be treated.

II.f.5 Complications of surgery and other medical care

When the admission is for treatment of a complication resulting from surgery or other medical care, the complication code is sequenced as the principal diagnosis/first listed code.

II.g Selection of secondary diagnoses

In most cases, more than one code is necessary to fully explain a health care encounter. Though a patient has an encounter for a primary reason (the principal/first listed diagnosis), the additional conditions or reasons for the encounter also need to be coded. These codes are referred to as secondary, additional or "other" diagnoses.

For reporting purposes the definition of "other diagnoses" is interpreted as additional conditions that affect patient care in terms of requiring:

> clinical evaluation; or
> therapeutic treatment; or
> diagnostic procedures; or
> extended length of hospital stay; or
> increased nursing care and/or monitoring.

The UHDDS item #11-b defines "Other Diagnoses" as "all conditions that coexist at the time of admission, that develop subsequently, or that affect the treatment received and/or the length of stay. Diagnoses that relate to an earlier episode which have no bearing on the current hospital stay are to be excluded." UHDDS definitions apply to inpatients in an acute care, short-term, hospital setting. This definition also applies to outpatient encounters.

If the attending physician has included a diagnosis in the final diagnostic statement, such as the discharge summary or the face sheet, it should ordinarily be coded, unless the condition does not meet the definition of "other diagnosis" listed above.

II.g.1 Previous conditions
Some physicians include in the diagnostic statement resolved conditions or diagnoses and status-post procedures from previous admission that have no bearing on the current stay. Such conditions are not to be reported and are coded only if required by hospital or physician office policy.

II.g.2 Abnormal test findings
Abnormal test findings (laboratory, x-ray, pathologic, and other diagnostic results) are not coded and reported unless the physician indicates their clinical significance. If the findings are outside the normal range and the physician has ordered other tests to evaluate the condition or prescribed treatment, it is appropriate to ask the physician whether the abnormal finding should be added.

If the abnormal test finding corresponds to a confirmed diagnosis it should not be coded in addition to the confirmed diagnosis.

Section III: Chapter-specific Coding Guidelines

In addition to the general coding guidelines, there are guidelines for specific diagnoses and/or conditions in the classification. Unless otherwise indicated, these guidelines apply to both inpatient and outpatient settings.

Chapter 1: Certain infectious and parasitic diseases

1.1 Human immunodeficiency virus [HIV] disease

The ICD-10-CM has four codes and one subcategory to classify the HIV virus:

Code B20, Human immunodeficiency virus [HIV] disease

Code Z21, Asymptomatic human immunodeficiency virus [HIV] infection status

Code R75, Inconclusive laboratory evidence of human immunodeficiency virus [HIV]

Code Z20.6, Exposure to HIV virus

Subcategory O98.7, HIV complicating pregnancy, childbirth, and the puerperium

Only code B20 is in Chapter 1. Codes Z21 and Z20.6 are located in Chapter 21, code R75 is located in Chapter 18. Subcategory O98.7 is located in Chapter 15.

Code B20, Human immunodeficiency virus [HIV] disease, is for use for symptomatic HIV patients. That is, patients who have or have had any of the opportunistic infections associated with the HIV virus. This code is synonymous with the terms Acquired immune deficiency syndrome (AIDS), and AIDS-related complex (ARC). Code Z21, Asymptomatic human immunodeficiency virus [HIV] infection status, is equivalent to the statement "HIV positive." Code Z21 is only for patients who are HIV positive but have never had any opportunistic infections. Once a patient has had a first opportunistic infection that patient is assigned code B20 from then on. They should never again be assigned a Z21 code, even if at a particular encounter no infection or HIV related condition is present. Codes B20 and Z21 should never appear on the same record.

Confirmation of HIV status does not require documentation of positive serology or culture for HIV. The physician's diagnostic statement that a patient is HIV positive, or has an HIV-related illness is sufficient.

Code R75 is for limited use for patients who have an inconclusive lab finding for HIV. It includes newborns of HIV positive mothers whose HIV status has not been confirmed. Code Z20.6, Exposure to HIV virus, is only for use in those instances when a patient believes he/she may have been exposed or come in contact with the HIV virus. See guideline 21.2.5 Contact/Exposure.

1.1.1 Sequencing of HIV codes

If a patient has a health care encounter for an HIV-related condition, code B20 should be sequenced first (principal/first listed code), followed by additional diagnosis codes for all reported HIV-related conditions. Codes for unrelated conditions should also be coded.

If an HIV patient has a health care encounter for an unrelated condition, such as trauma, the code for the unrelated condition should be sequenced first (principal/first listed code). B20 or Z21 should be added as an additional diagnosis. Any HIV-related diagnosis codes should also added, when applicable, to accompany the B20 code.

1.1.2 HIV in a pregnant patient

Codes from Chapter 15, Pregnancy, childbirth, and the puerperium, are always sequenced first on a medical record. Code O98.7-, HIV complicating pregnancy, childbirth, and the puerperium, should be used first, followed by the appropriate HIV code.

1.1.3 Encounter for testing for HIV

If the results of the test are positive follow the guidelines above. See guidelines 21.2.1 and 21.2.11 for coding of encounters for testing and counseling.

1.2 Sepsis

Sepsis refers to an infection due to any organism that triggers a systemic inflammatory response, the systemic inflammatory response syndrome (SIRS). All codes with sepsis in the title include the concept of SIRS. For cases of sepsis that do not result in any associated organ dysfunction, a single code for the type of sepsis should be used.

For other infections in which SIRS is present but sepsis is not in the code title, code R65.1, Systemic inflammatory response syndrome (SIRS), may also be assigned. For any infection, if associated organ dysfunction is present, a code from subcategory R65.2, Severe sepsis, should be used and the guidelines for coding of severe sepsis should be followed. See guideline 18.2 Severe sepsis and septic shock. Codes for sepsis and septic shock associated with abortion, ectopic pregnancy, and molar pregnancy are in Chapter 15. Code R65.1 and a code from R65.2 should not be used together on the same record.

The terms bacteremia and septicemia NOS are coded to R78.81. If a patient with a serious infection is documented to have septicemia the physician should be asked if the patient has sepsis. If any organ dysfunction is documented the physician should be asked if the patient has severe sepsis. Negative or inconclusive blood cultures do not preclude a diagnosis of sepsis in patients with clinical evidence of the condition.

The term urosepsis is a non-specific term. If a physician uses the term in a medical record he/she should be asked for which specific condition is the term being used.

1.3 Infectious agents as the cause of diseases classified to other chapters
Certain infections are classified in chapters other than Chapter 1 and no organism is identified as part of the infection code. In these instances, it is necessary to use an additional code from Chapter 1 to identify the organism. A code from category B95, Streptococcus, Staphylococcus, and Enterococcus as the cause of diseases classified to other chapters, B96, Other bacterial agents as the cause of diseases classified to other chapters, or B97, Viral agents as the cause of diseases classified to other chapters, is to be used as an additional code to identify the organism. An instructional note will be found at the infection code advising that an additional organism code is required.

1.4 Nosocomial infections
If a patient contract an infection while in the hospital, it is necessary to assign code Y95, Nosocomial condition, in addition to the infection code, to identify the infection as nosocomially acquired.

Chapter 2: Neoplasms

2.1 Neoplasm Table
Chapter 2 of the ICD-10-CM contains the codes for most benign and all malignant neoplasms. Certain benign neoplasms, such as prostatic adenomas, are found in the specific body system chapters. To properly code a neoplasm, it is necessary to determine from the record if the neoplasm is benign, in-situ, malignant, or, of uncertain histologic behavior. If malignant, any secondary (metastatic) sites should also be determined.

The Index for the ICD-10-CM has a separate Table of Neoplasms. It should be used to select the correct code(s). If the histology (cell type) of the neoplasm is documented, that term should be referenced first, in the main section of the Index, rather than going immediately to the Neoplasm Table, in order to determine which column in the Neoplasm Table is appropriate. For example, if the documentation indicates "adenocarcinoma," refer to the term in the Index to review the entries under this term and the instructional note to "see also neoplasm, by site, malignant." The Neoplasm Table provides the proper code based on the histology of the neoplasm and the site. It is important to select a code from the proper column of the Neoplasm Table that corresponds to the histology of the neoplasm. The Tabular List should then be referenced to verify that the correct code has been selected and that a more specific site code does not exist.

2.2 Use of pathology report
A malignant neoplasm code should not be assigned at the time of initial diagnosis without a pathology report on the record confirming the histologic type of the neoplasm. If the pathology report is not on the record, confirmation of the diagnosis by the attending physician should be documented. A pathology report is not required for confirmed cases, such as encounters for chemotherapy or radiation therapy.

2.3 Morphology codes

Though the Neoplasm Table provides codes based on the histologic type, it only distinguishes between in-situ, benign, malignant or "of uncertain behavior." A secondary morphology code is needed to specifically identify the histologic type of the tumor. A morphology code should be included on a medical record that has a neoplasm diagnosis whenever possible. The morphology codes are found in a separate section of the classification. The proper morphology code can be located in the Index under the term for the histology of the neoplasm.

2.4 Neoplasms of uncertain behavior versus neoplasms of unspecified behavior

A neoplasm of uncertain behavior (Categories D37-D48) is one which after histologic examination is unable to be classified as malignant or benign. The pathologic interpretation is that the cell type cannot be determined.

A neoplasm of unspecified behavior (Category D49) code is only used when there is no documentation in the record indicating the nature of the neoplasm. The unspecified behavior code should not be used if any histologic examination has been made of the excised or biopsied tissue.

2.5 Sequencing of neoplasm codes

If the reason for the encounter is for diagnosis of a suspicious lump, skin lesion, or other indication that a malignancy might be present assign the code for the sign or symptom until confirmation of the diagnosis is made. At the time of coding, if confirmation of a malignancy has been made for an outpatient visit, the neoplasm code should be assigned.

If the reason for the encounter is for treatment of the primary neoplasm, assign the neoplasm as the principal/first listed diagnosis. The primary site is to be sequenced first, followed by any metastatic sites.

When an encounter is for a primary malignancy with metastasis and treatment is directed toward the metastatic (secondary) site(s) only, the metastatic site(s) is designated as the principal/first listed diagnosis. The primary malignancy is coded as an additional code.

When an encounter is for management of a complication associated with the malignancy, such as dehydration, and the treatment is only for the complication, the complication is coded first, followed by the appropriate code(s) for the malignancy. An exception to this is anemia due to a neoplasm. Code D63.0, Anemia in neoplastic disease, is a manifestation (secondary) code. Coding conventions require that it be sequenced after the underlying neoplasm code.

When an encounter is for a pathological fracture due to a malignancy, if the focus of treatment is the fracture, a code from subcategory M84.5, Pathological fracture of bone in neoplastic disease, should be sequenced first, followed by the code for the malignancy. If the focus of treatment is the neoplasm with an associated pathological fracture, the neoplasm code should be sequenced first, followed by a code from M84.5 for the pathological fracture. The "code also" note at

M84.5 provides this sequencing instruction.

When an encounter is for pain management due to the malignancy, the pain code, R52.02, R52.12, or, R52.22 should be sequenced first, followed by the appropriate neoplasm code(s). See guideline 18.3 Encounter for pain management.

When the encounter is for treatment of a complication resulting from a surgical procedure performed for the treatment of a malignancy, designate the complication as the principal/first-listed diagnosis if treatment is directed at resolving the complication.

When a primary malignancy has been previously excised or eradicated from its site and there is no further treatment directed to that site and there is no evidence of any existing primary malignancy, a code from category Z85, Personal history of primary and secondary malignant neoplasm, should be used to indicate the former site of the malignancy. Any mention of extension, invasion, or metastasis to another site(s) is coded as a secondary malignant neoplasm to the metastatic site(s). The secondary site may be the principal/first listed with the Z85 code used as a secondary code. See guideline 21.2.12 History (of).

When a primary malignancy has been excised but further treatment, such as an additional surgery, radiation therapy or chemotherapy is directed to that site, the primary malignancy code, not the Z85 code should be used until treatment is completed.

2.6 Cancer in a pregnant patient
Codes from chapter 15, Pregnancy, childbirth, and the puerperium, are always sequenced first on a medical record. A code from subcategory O94.1-, Malignant neoplasm complicating pregnancy, childbirth, and the puerperium, should be used first, followed by the appropriate code from Chapter 2 to indicate the type of neoplasm.

2.7 Malignant neoplasm without specification of site
Code C80, Malignant neoplasm without specification of site, equates to Cancer, unspecified. It is also for disseminated cancer for which no primary site is found. This code should only be used when no determination can be made as to the primary site of a malignancy. It should not be used in place of assigning codes for the primary site and for all known secondary sites.

2.8 Encounters for chemotherapy and radiation therapy
When an encounter involves the surgical removal of a neoplasm, primary or secondary site, followed by chemotherapy or radiation treatment, the neoplasm code should be assigned as the principal/first-listed diagnosis.

If an encounter is solely for the administration of chemotherapy or radiation therapy code Z51.0, Encounter for radiotherapy session, or Z51.1, Encounter for chemotherapy session for neoplasm, should be the principal/first listed code. If a patient receives both chemotherapy and radiation therapy both codes should be listed, in either order of sequence.

When an encounter is for the purpose of radiotherapy or chemotherapy and the patient develops complications such as uncontrolled nausea and vomiting or dehydration, the principal/first-listed code remains the radiation therapy or chemotherapy code. The complications of the treatment should be added as additional codes.

When an encounter is to determine the extent of the malignancy, or for a procedure to treat the malignancy, the primary malignancy or appropriate metastatic site is designated as the principal/first-listed diagnosis, even if chemotherapy or radiotherapy is administered.

When an encounter is for management of the complication of chemotherapy or radiation therapy, and the only treatment is for the complication, the complication is sequenced first followed by the appropriate code(s) for the malignancy.

Due to the potentially toxic nature of many chemotherapy agents certain tests may be performed prior to the administration of chemotherapy as well as during the course of the chemotherapy treatment. The malignancy should be coded as the principal diagnosis for encounters for these tests. The code for long-term (current) use of drug, Z79.82, should be used as a secondary code if the test is being done during the course of chemotherapy treatment.

2.9 Endocrine therpy
Endocrine therapy, such a Tamoxifen, may be given prophylactically, for women at high-risk of developing breast cancer. It may also be given during cancer treatment as well as following treatment to help prevent recurrence. The use of endocrine therapy does not affect the guidelines for coding of neoplasms.

Chapter 3:   Diseases of the blood and blood-forming organs and certain disorders involving the immune mechanism

3.1 Intraoperative and postprocedural hematologic and immune system complications- see guideline 19.3.5.4. Complications of care within body system chapters

Chapter 4: Endocrine, nutritional, and metabolic diseases

4.1 Diabetes mellitus
The Diabetes mellitus (DM) codes are combination codes that include the type of DM, the body system affected, and the complications affecting that body system. As many codes within a particular category as are necessary to describe all of the complications of the disease may be used. They should be sequenced based on the reason for a particular visit.

There are 6 DM categories in the ICD-10-CM:
E08, Diabetes mellitus due to underlying condition
E09, Drug or chemical induced diabetes mellitus
E10, Type 1 diabetes mellitus

E11, Type 2 diabetes mellitus
E13, Other specified diabetes mellitus
E14, Unspecified diabetes mellitus

Definitions for the types of DM are a component of the Includes notes under each DM category in the Tabular List. The concepts of insulin and non-insulin requiring diabetes mellitus are not a component of the DM categories in the ICD-10-CM. An additional code, Z79.5, Long-term (current) use of insulin, may be added to identify the use of insulin for diabetic management for categories E08-E09 and E11-E14.

Sequencing of diabetes codes from categories E08 and E09 are based on the convention found at each category. Categories E08 and E09 have a "code first" note indicating that the diabetes code is to be sequenced after the underlying condition, drug or chemical, that is responsible for the diabetes. Codes from categories E10-E14 are sequenced first, followed by codes for any additional complications outside these categories, if needed.

4.1.1 Diabetes mellitus in a pregnant patient
Codes from Chapter 15, Pregnancy, childbirth, and the puerperium, are always sequenced first on a medical record. A pregnant woman with pre-existing DM should be assigned a code from category O24, Diabetes mellitus in pregnancy, childbirth, and the puerperium, first, followed by the appropriate diabetes code from Chapter 4. For women who develop diabetes during pregnancy, see guideline 15.7, Gestational diabetes.

4.1.2 Diabetic patients who receive an organ(s) transplant
Patients who receive a new pancreas for treatment of their DM may no longer require insulin or other care for their DM, but pre-existing complications from the DM may still exist after transplant. Codes from the DM categories are still applicable to describe the complications in such cases. A transplant status code should be used with the diabetes code in these cases.

4.2 Intraoperative and postprocedural endocrine system complications- See guideline 19.3.5.4 Complications of care within the body system chapters.

Chapter 5: Mental and behavioral disorders

5.1 ICD-10-CM and DSM-IV-TR
The codes in Chapter 5 parallel, in most cases, the codes found in the Diagnostic and Statistical Manual of Mental Disorders, fourth edition, text revision (DSM-IV TR) published by the American Psychiatric Association. For definitions of the psychiatric terms and conditions used in this chapter, reference the DSM-IV TR. Selection of the proper code from Chapter 5 should be based solely on the terminology and documentation found in the medical record.

5.2 Alcohol and drug abuse and dependence
The drug and alcohol codes are multiaxial, combination codes that identify the substance, the

type of use, abuse or dependence, and the complications and manifestations caused by the substance. The category level is the substance, such as, alcohol (F10) and other types of drugs, (F11-F19), including nicotine, (F17). The 4th character axis distinguishes abuse or dependence. The 5th and 6th characters indicate the complication, such as withdrawal or delusions. The types of complications and manifestations at the 5th and 6th character are specific to the type of drug.

Multiple codes from a single category from categories F10-F19 may be used together, if a patient has multiple complications from a single substance. Multiple codes from different categories from F10-F19 may be used together, if a patient has used more than one substance and has multiple complications associated with the use of the substances.

An additional code from category Y90, Evidence of alcohol involvement determined by blood alcohol level, should be used with a code from F10, Alcohol-related disorders, if the patient's blood alcohol level is recorded. A code from Y90 should be recorded only once, at the initial blood alcohol level reading.

Codes from the poisoning and toxic effects section of Chapter 19 (T40, T51) should be used in conjunction with the F10-F19 codes if a patient has an acute alcohol or drug poisoning or overdose, even if the patient is dependent on alcohol or drugs. See guideline 19.3.2 Poisonings, toxic effects, adverse effects and underdosing.

5.3 Dementia with behavioral disturbance
Category F02, Dementia in other diseases classified elsewhere, is a manifestation category that is for use with codes for specific types of dementia, such as Alzheimer's disease (G30). The code for the specific type of dementia is sequenced first, followed by the appropriate code from category F02. The code from category F02 indicates whether the dementia has an associated behavioral disturbance.

Chapter 6: Diseases of nervous system

6.1 Dominant/nondominant side
For patients with hemiplegia and other paralytic syndromes the side involved is important in determining potential for recovery. Patients whose dominant side is affected will have a more difficult time with rehabilitation than patients whose nondominant side is affected. Generally, the patient's dominance is recorded in the initial history and physical. If there is reference to a patient being right-handed or left-handed this indicates dominance. Dominance is present in both the upper and lower limbs.

Codes from category G81, Hemiplegia and hemiparesis, and subcategories, G83.1, Monoplegia of lower limb, G83.2, Monoplegia of upper limb, and G83.3, Monoplegia, unspecified, have a final character for dominant and nondominant side. Should this information not be available in the record, the default should be dominant. For ambidextrous patients, the default should also be dominant.

6.2 Parkinson's disease

There are 2 categories in the ICD-10-CM for Parkinson's disease, G20, Parkinson's disease and G21, Secondary parkinsonism. G20 is the code for primary Parkinson's disease. It is the default code for the condition.

G21, Secondary parkinsonism, is a result of another condition such as an encephalitis or poisoning. The symptoms of Parkinson's disease develop secondary to the initial condition. The sequencing of a code from G21 is based on the conventions found at the G21 codes.

The shakes and tremors associated with Parkinson's disease are also symptoms of a form of dementia, dementia with Lewy bodies (G31.83). The term dementia with Parkinsonism is included under code G31.83. G31.83 is excluded from G21.

6.3 Dementia

Two codes are required for dementia. First the dementia code, followed by a secondary code from category F02 for the behavioral component of the dementia. See guideline 5.3 Dementia with behavioral disturbance.

Cases of dementia are often diagnosed strictly by the symptoms and behavior of the patient. For certain types of dementia confirmation of the diagnosis can only be made at autopsy. For this reason physicians often document probable or suspected dementia. Dementia is one group of conditions where it is acceptable to code the condition even if it is stated as probable or suspected.

6.4 Intraoperative and postprocedural nervous system complications- See guideline 19.3.5.4 Complications of care within the body system chapters.

Chapter 7: Diseases of the eye and adnexa

7.1 Laterality

For most of the categories in Chapter 7 there are codes for right eye, left eye, and bilateral. In cases where a code does not provide a designation for which eye is involved, that condition is always bilateral. In cases where a bilateral code is not provided the condition is always unilateral.

7.2 Intraoperative and postprocedural ophthalmologic complications- See guideline 19.3.5.4 Complications of care within the body system chapters.

Chapter 8: Diseases of the ear and mastoid process

8.1 Intraoperative and postprocedural auditory system complications- See guideline 19.3.5.4.
Complications of care within the body system chapters.

Chapter 9: Diseases of circulatory system

9.1 Rheumatic heart disease
The default for the coding of certain heart valve disease is rheumatic. However, if there is no
documentation in the medical record that a patient has had rheumatic fever, the non-rheumatic
code should be assigned.

9.2 Hypertension

9.2.1 Hypertensive heart disease
The codes in category I11, Hypertensive heart disease, are combination codes that include both
hypertension and heart disease. The "Includes" note at I11 specifies the conditions that are
included with I11. If a patient has both a condition listed in the "Includes" note and hypertension
then a code from I11 should be used, not individual codes for hypertension and heart disease. No
causal relationship needs to be documented.

The final character of the codes identifies with and without heart failure. The default is without
heart failure. For code I11.0, Hypertensive heart disease with heart failure, a secondary code
from category I50, Heart failure, is required to identify the type of heart failure.

9.2.2 Hypertensive renal disease
The codes in category I12, Hypertensive renal disease, are combination codes that include both
hypertension and renal disease. The "Includes" note at I12 specifies the conditions that are
included with I12. If a patient has both a condition listed in the "Includes" note and hypertension
then a code from I12 should be used, not individual codes for hypertension and renal disease. No
causal relationship needs to be documented.

The final character of the codes identifies with or without chronic renal failure. The default is
without chronic renal failure. If a patient has hypertension with both acute and chronic renal
failure, an additional code for the acute renal failure is required.

9.2.3 Hypertensive heart and renal disease
The codes in category I13, Hypertensive heart and renal disease, are combination codes that
include hypertension, heart disease and renal disease. The Includes note at I13 specifies that the
conditions included at I11 and I12 make up I13. If a patient has hypertension, heart disease and
renal disease then a code from I13 should be used, not individual codes for hypertension, heart
disease and renal disease, or codes from I11 or I12.

For patients with heart failure a secondary code from category I50, Heart failure, is required. For patients with both acute and chronic renal failure an additional code for acute renal failure is required.

9.2.4 Hypertensive retinopathy
Code H35.0, Hypertensive retinopathy, may be used alone, or with code I10, Essential (primary) hypertension, to include the systemic hypertension. If both codes are used the sequencing is based on the reason for the encounter.

9.2.5 Secondary hypertension
Secondary hypertension is due to an underlying condition but category I15, Secondary hypertension, is not a manifestation (paired) category. Two codes are required when assigning a code from I15, one to identify the underlying etiology and one from category I15 to identify the hypertension. The sequencing of the codes is based on the reason for the encounter.

9.2.6 Hypertension, controlled
This diagnostic statement usually refers to an existing state of hypertension under control by therapy. Assign code I10.

9.2.7 Hypertension, uncontrolled
Uncontrolled hypertension may refer to untreated hypertension or hypertension not responding to current therapeutic regimen. In either case, it should be coded as hypertension.

9.2.8 Elevated blood pressure
For a statement of elevated blood pressure without further specificity, assign code R03.0, Elevated blood-pressure reading, without diagnosis of hypertension, rather than code I10. R03.0 is also for use for a single elevated blood pressure reading or for transient elevated blood pressure.

9.3 Atherosclerotic coronary artery disease and angina
ICD-10-CM has combination codes for atherosclerotic heart disease with angina pectoris. The subcategories for these codes are I25.11, Atherosclerotic heart disease of native coronary artery with angina pectoris and I25.7, Atherosclerosis of coronary artery bypass graft(s) and coronary artery of transplanted heart with angina pectoris. The codes identify the type of angina.

When using a combination code it is not necessary to use an additional angina pectoris code. A causal relationship can be assumed in a patient with both atherosclerosis and angina pectoris, unless the documentation indicates the angina is due to something other than the atherosclerosis. The angina does not have to be documented to be due to the specified occluded artery.

If a patient with coronary artery disease is admitted due to an acute myocardial infarction (AMI), the AMI should be sequenced before the coronary artery disease. See guideline 9.4 Initial and subsequent acute myocardial infarction (AMI)

9.4 Initial and subsequent acute myocardial infarction (AMI)

The ICD-10-CM has two categories for acute myocardial infarction, I21, Acute myocardial infarction and I22, Subsequent acute myocardial infarction. The I21 is for all cases of initial myocardial infarction. A code from I21 is to be used from onset of the AMI until 4 weeks following onset. The 4 week period is considered the length of time needed for healing.

A code from I22 is to be used if a patient who has suffered an AMI has a new AMI within the 4 week time frame of the initial MI. A code from category I22, Subsequent myocardial infarction, must be used in conjunction with a code from category I21, Acute myocardial infarction.

The sequencing of the I22 and I21 codes depends on the circumstances of the encounter. Should a patient who is in the hospital due to an AMI have a subsequent AMI while still in the hospital, the I21 would be sequenced first as the reason for admission with the I22 code sequenced as a secondary code. Should a patient have a subsequent AMI after discharge for care of an initial AMI and the reason for admission is the subsequent AMI, the I22 code should be sequenced first followed by the I21. The I21 must accompany the I22 to show the site of the initial AMI and to indicate that the patient is still within the 4 week time frame of healing from the initial AMI.

When both an AMI and atherosclerotic coronary artery disease are documented in a medical record the AMI is to be sequenced first followed by a code for the coronary artery disease. This sequencing is based on the acute life-threatening condition being the principal reason for admission. Though treatment of the AMI is directed at relieving the occlusion caused by the underlying coronary artery disease, the majority of adults have some amount of atherosclerotic plaque in their coronary arteries. It is only when the atherosclerosis is severe enough to obstruct blood flow to the heart that an AMI occurs, necessitating immediate attention. When coding atherosclerotic coronary artery disease with an AMI the appropriate coronary artery disease combination code for "with unstable angina" should be used.

9.5 Cardiac arrest

There are three codes under category I46, I46.2, Cardiac arrest due to underlying cardiac condition, I46.8, Cardiac arrest due to other underlying condition, and I46.9, Cardiac arrest, cause unspecified.

I46.9, Cardiac arrest, cause unspecified, is acceptable as a principal diagnosis only if the patient expires or is discharged within 24 hours of admission to the hospital or the emergency department and no determination is made as to the cause of the cardiac arrest. Though a cardiac arrest qualifies as an emergent, life-threatening condition, it is considered a non-specific principal diagnosis. Code I46.9 should not be used as a secondary diagnosis unless the cause of the arrest is undocumented.

I46.2, Cardiac arrest due to underlying cardiac condition, and I46.8, Cardiac arrest due to other underlying condition, may be used as secondary diagnoses when a patient with an underlying condition suffers an arrest while under care for the underlying condition. These codes should never be used as the principal diagnosis since their use indicates that the underlying cause is known.

Should attempts be made to resuscitate a patient who suffers a cardiac arrest a code from I46 should be used regardless of whether the resuscitation is successful or not. The procedure code on the record will indicate that a resuscitation attempt was performed.

9.6 Cerebrovascular occlusion and stenosis and cerebral infarction
There are three categories in ICD-10-CM for occlusion and stenosis of the precerebral and cerebral arteries that incorporate the presence or absence of cerebral infarction. Category I63, Cerebral infarction, identifies the site and type of the infarct at the 4th character level. Category I65, Occlusion and stenosis of precerebral arteries, not resulting in cerebral infarction, and Category I66, Occlusion and stenosis of cerebral arteries, not resulting in cerebral infarction, are for use when there is evidence of obstruction of a vessel but there is no resulting evidence of an infarct.

A code from I65 and I66 should not be used with a code from I63 of the same artery. A code from I65 and I66 may be used with a code from I63 if a patient has both an infarction of one artery and occlusion of other arteries. It is often difficult to determine the site of a cerebral infarction in a patient with extensive cerebrovascular disease. Documentation in the record and consultation with the physician, if necessary, is required to determine the correct code or codes from the I63, I65, and I66 categories. Code I63.9, Cerebral infarction, unspecified, may be used if an infarction is documented but no artery is specified.

9.7 Stroke, not specified as hemorrhage or infarction
Code I64, Stroke, not specified as hemorrhage or infarction, is the generic, non-specific code for a cerebrovascular accident (CVA). It is only for use in limited circumstances when no documentation is available indicating the type of stroke. When documentation exists, a code for a cerebral infarction or hemorrhage should be used, not I64. See guideline 9.8 Sequelae of cerebrovascular disease.

9.8 Sequelae of cerebrovascular disease
Category I69, Sequelae of cerebrovascular disease, is for use to classify the complications of intracerebral hemorrhage and infarction. Codes from I69 can be used as soon after the initial cerebrovascular accident as sequelae appear. Codes under I69 include the site and type of the CVA at the subcategory level, the fifth character identifies the sequelae and the 6th character identifies the side of the body affected. As many codes as are necessary to identify all of the sequelae may be used.

A code from I69 may be used in conjunction with a current cerebral hemorrhage or infarction code if a patient has a current hemorrhage or infarction of either the same site or of a different site at the same time as the sequelae.

9.9 Intraoperative and postprocedural circulatory system complications- See guideline 19.3.5.4 Complications of care within the body system chapters.

Chapter 10: Diseases of respiratory system

10.1 Chronic obstructive pulmonary disease (COPD)
The ICD-10-CM category for chronic bronchitis is J42, for emphysema J43, for chronic obstructive pulmonary disease (COPD), J44, and for asthma, J45.

If a patient has a single condition, either chronic bronchitis, emphysema or asthma, a single code from the appropriate category should be used.

For a patient who has a combination of chronic obstructive lung problems, a single code from category J44 is usually appropriate. The following combination of conditions, stated as such in the medical record, are included under category J44:
    asthma with chronic obstructive pulmonary disease
    chronic bronchitis with airway obstruction
    chronic bronchitis with emphysema
    chronic emphysematous bronchitis
    chronic obstructive asthma
    chronic obstructive bronchitis
    chronic obstructive tracheobronchitis
Only these combinations are included in category J44 . Any combinations not included must be coded with individual codes.

The codes in category J44, Other chronic obstructive pulmonary disease, indicate whether a patient has an uncomplicated case, an acute exacerbation or a co-existing acute lower respiratory infection. The code for the acute lower respiratory infection takes precedence over the acute exacerbation. If the infection is a pneumonia or influenza, a secondary code for the type of pneumonia or the influenza is also needed.

10.2 Nosocomial respiratory infections
If a patient contract a respiratory infection while in the hospital, it is necessary to assign code Y95, Nosocomial condition, in addition to the infection code, to identify the infection as nosocomially acquired.

10.3 Intraoperative and postprocedural respiratory system complications- See guideline 19.3.5.4 Complications of care within the body system chapters.

Chapter 11: Diseases of digestive system

11.1 Ulcers
All of the codes under ulcer categories, K25, Gastric ulcer, K26, Duodenal ulcer, K27, Peptic ulcer, site unspecified, and K28, Gastrojejunal ulcer, have combinations codes that identify complications of the ulcer, (bleeding, and perforation). No secondary complication codes are needed when using one of the combination codes for ulcers. Multiple codes from each category may be used if a patient has multiple complications.

11.2 Crohn's disease/ulcerative colitis
The codes under subcategories K50, Crohn's disease, and K51, Ulcerative colitis, identify a single complication of the conditions. Should a patient have multiple complications, multiple codes from K50 or K51 may be used to identify each of the complications.

11.3 Intraoperative and postprocedural digestive system complications- See guideline 19.3.5.4 Complications of care within the body system chapters.

Chapter 12: Diseases of the skin and subcutaneous tissue

12.1 Dermatology codes and use of an external cause
For categories L56, Other acute skin changes due to ultraviolet radiation, and L57, Skin changes due to chronic exposure to nonionizing radiation, a secondary external cause code identifying the source of the exposure should be used.

For codes L56.0, Drug phototoxic response, and L56.1, Drug photoallergic response, and all other codes that identify a dermatologic condition due to a drug or chemical, a code from categories T36-T50, Poisoning and adverse effects of drugs, medicaments and biological substances, and T51-T65, Toxic effects of substances chiefly nonmedicinal as to source, is to be sequenced first, to identify the drug or chemical, followed by the dermatology code. See guideline 19.3.2 Poisoning, toxic effects, adverse effects and underdosing.

No external cause code is needed for category L55, Sunburn.

12.2 Decubitus ulcers and non-decubitus chronic ulcers of lower limb codes
The codes in categories L89, Decubitus ulcer, and L97, Non-decubitus chronic ulcer of lower limb, not elsewhere classified, contain a great deal of detail. The 5th character of the codes identifies the specific site of the ulcer. The 6th character identifies the depth of the ulcer. When assigning a code for these ulcers it is important to review the record thoroughly to verify both the site and severity of the ulcer. For multiple ulcers of the same site, it is only necessary to assign a code for the most severe ulcer.

The sequencing instructions at categories L89 and L97 differ slightly from the standard conventions. Decubitus ulcers may occur at multiple sites. A decubitus ulcer that has become very serious and does not respond to treatment may be the reason for admission to a hospital. The decubitus ulcer should be the principal diagnosis if it is the reason for admission. Secondary codes for the other health problems associated with the decubitus ulcer should also be assigned.

Generally, an underlying condition is responsible for a non-decubitus ulcer of the lower limb (L97.-). Any condition that reduces blood flow to the legs may cause a lower limb ulcer. The same condition may also prevent healing of the ulcer even with aggressive treatment. When the underlying condition is known, the underlying condition should be sequenced before the ulcer. Atherosclerosis of the lower extremities and diabetes mellitus are commonly the underlying conditions responsible. Combination codes for atherosclerosis of the lower extremities and diabetes mellitus include lower extremity ulcers. A code from L97 to specify the site and depth of the ulcer is needed with the combination code for the underlying condition. In some cases no underlying cause is documented to be responsible for the ulcer. In such cases a code from L97 may be principal or first listed. The instructional note at L97 indicates that the "code first" note is applicable only when an underlying condition is documented.

Both decubitus and non-decubitus ulcers may become so severe that gangrene sets in at the site of the ulcer. For cases of gangrene resulting from a skin ulcer, the gangrene should be sequenced first, followed by the code for the ulcer. Gangrene is necrosis of the tissue. When gangrene is present, the primary focus of treatment is to remove the gangrene, usually with debridement or amputation of the affected area. The "code first" note at categories L89 and L97 instructs that gangrene is to be sequenced before the ulcer. This note applies only if gangrene is present.

12.3 Intraoperative and postprocedural dermatologic complications- See guideline 19.3.5.4 Complications of care within the body system chapters.

Chapter 13: Diseases of the musculoskeletal system and connective tissue

13.1 Site and laterality
Most of the codes within Chapter 13 have site and laterality designations. The site represents either the bone, joint or the muscle involved. For some conditions where more than one bone, joint or muscle is usually involved, there is a multiple site code available. For categories where no multiple site code is provided and more than one bone, joint or muscle is involved, multiple codes should be used to indicate the different sites involved.

The site designations for the limbs are upper arm, lower arm, upper leg and lower leg, (humerus, radius and ulna, femur, tibia and fibula). When a condition is described as of the arm or leg, without indicating upper or lower, then the code for upper arm or lower leg should be used.

For certain conditions, the bone may be affected at the upper or lower end, (e.g., avascular necrosis of bone, M87, Osteoporosis, M80, M81). Though the portion of the bone affected may be at the joint, the site designation will be the bone, not the joint.

13.2 Acute/chronic/recurrent musculoskeletal conditions

Many of the conditions in chapter 13 are a result of previous injury or trauma to a site, or are recurrent conditions. Any current, acute injury should be coded to the appropriate injury code. Bone, joint or muscle conditions that are the result of a healed injury are usually found in chapter 13. Recurrent bone, joint or muscle conditions are also usually found in chapter 13. If it is difficult to determine from the documentation in the record which code is best to describe a condition, confer with the physician.

13.3 Osteoporosis

There are 2 categories for osteoporosis, M80, Osteoporosis with current pathologic fracture, and M81, Osteoporosis without current pathologic fracture. Osteoporosis is a systemic condition, meaning that all bones of the musculoskeletal system are affected. For this reason, site codes are not provided for codes M81.0, Postmenopausal osteoporosis without current pathological fracture, and M81.8, Other osteoporosis without current pathological fracture.

M81 is for use for patients with osteoporosis who do not currently have a pathologic fracture due to the osteoporosis, even if they have had a fracture in the past. For patients with a history of osteoporosis fractures, status code Z87.31, Personal history of osteoporosis fracture, should accompany the code from M81.

Category M80 is for a patient who has a current pathologic fracture at the time of the encounter. The codes under M80 identify the site of the fracture. A pathologic fracture code, not a traumatic fracture code, should be used for any patient with known osteoporosis who suffers a fracture, even if the patient had a minor fall or trauma, if that fall or trauma would not usually break a normal, healthy bone.

13.4 Intraoperative and postprocedural musculoskeletal system complications- See guideline 19.3.5.4 Complications of care within the body system chapters.

13.5 Pathologic fracture in neoplastic disease- See guideline 2.5 Sequencing of neoplasm codes.

Chapter 14: Diseases of the genitourinary system

14.1 Renal failure

There are two categories for renal failure in ICD-10-CM, N17, Acute renal failure (ARF), N18, Chronic renal failure (CRF), and code N19, Unspecified renal failure. N19 is a nonspecific code that should rarely be used in the inpatient setting. Uremia NOS is included under N19. If the term uremia is documented in a medical record, the physician should be asked for a more precise diagnosis.

ARF, though a serious condition that is life-threatening if left untreated, is generally a result of an underlying condition that is affecting kidney function. Correction of the underlying condition restores normal kidney function. The "code also" note at N17 instructs that ARF may be either a principal diagnosis or secondary code. The diagnosis of ARF indicates that the underlying condition is causing a serious problem and requires immediate attention. Sequencing is based on the severity of the underlying condition and the primary focus of treatment. ARF is always the result of another condition so, regardless of the sequencing it should never be the single condition coded on a record. A code from N17 should always have an accompanying code for the causal condition.

Dehydration and urinary obstruction are two common conditions that may cause ARF. Generally, rehydrating the patient and relieving the obstruction is adequate to correct the ARF. For these types of conditions the ARF should be sequenced before the underlying condition if it is the focus of treatment. Otherwise, the underlying condition should be sequenced first.

When the underlying condition is serious in itself and treatment is directed at the underlying condition, the underlying condition should be sequenced before ARF. An example of this is severe sepsis. It is life-threatening and treatment is directed at correcting all of the organ dysfunctions for which it is responsible. ARF is just one of many serious complications that may result from severe sepsis. Severe sepsis should be coded before any of the organ dysfunction codes, including ARF.

CRF is a non-reversible malfunctioning of the kidneys that results from conditions such as chronic hypertension and diabetes mellitus or from certain drugs or chemicals that damage the kidneys. Treatment for CRF is generally regular hemodialysis or peritoneal dialysis. CRF is not generally a reason for an inpatient admission except for patients admitted for kidney and other organ transplant. For patients receiving dialysis or care associated with dialysis in any setting, a code from category Z49, Encounter for care involving renal dialysis, should be the first listed code followed by a code from N18.

When a combination code exists for a condition that includes the CRF, such as diabetes mellitus with renal complications or hypertensive renal disease a second code from N18 is not needed.

14.2 Infertility
Codes for male infertility (N46) are not for use on a female record, even if a woman is receiving assisted reproductive therapy due to male partner infertility. Code Z31.81, Encounter for male factor infertility in female patient, is for use on a female record for these situations. Additional codes may be used in conjunction with Z31.81 to fully describe the encounter for assisted reproductive therapy.

14.3 Hyperplasia of prostate
The codes in category N40, Hyperplasia of prostate, are combination codes that include both the condition of the prostate and the associated complications, such as obstruction and hematuria. When using a code from category N40, it is not necessary to add secondary codes for the associated complications that are included in the codes.

14.4 Hypertensive renal disease- See guideline 9.2.2 Hypertensive renal disease.

14.5 Intraoperative and postprocedural genitourinary system complications- See guideline 19.3.5.4 Complications of care within the body system chapters.

Chapter 15: Pregnancy, childbirth and the puerperium

15.1 General Chapter 15 Guidelines
Codes from Chapter 15 take sequencing precedence over codes from all other chapters. Regardless of any other condition a pregnant woman may have, the appropriate obstetric (OB) code is to be sequenced first, followed by codes for the co-existing conditions.

Code Z33.1, Pregnant state, incidental, should only be used in rare instances. Any co-existing condition occurring during pregnancy should be considered a complication of the pregnancy unless expressly documented in the record that it is not affecting the pregnancy.

There are combination OB codes for conditions from all other chapters of the classification, including neoplasms and trauma. The OB combination code may not include as much detail as the code from the body system chapter. "Use additional code" notes are found at many Chapter 15 categories indicating that a secondary code is needed to provide more detail on the condition(s) from other chapters that are affecting the pregnancy.

Codes from Chapter 15 are for use only on the maternal record, never on the record of a newborn.

Codes in Chapter 15 represent only the diagnosis or reason for encounter. All procedures resulting from conditions found in Chapter 15, including delivery, must be indicated with a procedure code.

15.2 Sequencing of obstetric (OB) codes
The first OB code assigned should be based on the most significant reason for the encounter. For encounters when no delivery occurs, the first assigned diagnosis should correspond to the most significant complication of the pregnancy, which necessitated the encounter. Should more than one complication exist, all of which are treated or monitored, any of the complications codes may be sequenced first.

When a delivery occurs, the principal diagnosis should correspond to the main circumstances or complication of the delivery.

In encounters with a cesarean delivery, the selection of the principal diagnosis should correspond to the reason the cesarean delivery was performed, unless the reason for the encounter was unrelated to the condition resulting in the cesarean delivery.

15.3 Trimesters

The majority of codes in Chapter 15, beginning with category O09, have a final character indicating the trimester of pregnancy. The timeframes for the trimesters are indicated at the beginning of the chapter. If no trimester character is provided for a specific code in a category, it is because the condition always occurs in a specific trimester, or the trimester is not applicable, such as a postpartum condition. An example of this is gestational diabetes. It only occurs in late pregnancy. Certain codes have characters for only certain trimesters, not all three, because the condition does not occur in all trimesters, but it may occur in more than just one.

Each category that includes codes for trimester has a code for "unspecified trimester." The "unspecified trimester" code is never to be used, unless it is impossible to determine the trimester of the pregnancy from the documentation in the record.

For a patient who enters the hospital for complications of pregnancy and remains in the hospital for antepartum complications, delivery, and postpartum complications, it is acceptable to use the final character that corresponds to the trimester of the occurrence of the complication. It is acceptable to use codes indicating different trimesters of pregnancy as well as postpartum on the same record.

15.4   Complications of ectopic pregnancy, miscarriage and other abnormal products of
        conception

Complications of ectopic pregnancies, category O00, hydatidiform mole, category O01, other abnormal products of conception, category O02 and spontaneous abortion, category O03, require a code from category O08, Complications following ectopic and molar pregnancy to identify the complication. Should an encounter be for the complication itself, after the initial encounter for the pregnancy, a code from O08 should be the first listed code with no code from O00-O03.

Any procedure required for these conditions, such as the removal of retained products of conception, requires a procedure code from the appropriate procedure classification.

15.5 Multiple gestations

Chapter 15 has extensions for multiple gestations. An extension must be added to any code from Chapter 15 in which there is a multiple gestation pregnancy, indicating which fetus is affected by the particular condition being coded. Each fetus must be given an extension designation and this designation must be documented in the record so that the appropriate code(s) may be assigned consistently to the correct fetus.

An ectopic pregnancy (category O00) occurring with an intrauterine pregnancy is considered a multiple gestation. Both the ectopic pregnancy and the intrauterine pregnancy should be assigned an extension. Any complication code for the ectopic pregnancy (category O08) should have the same extension as the code from O00. All codes for the intrauterine pregnancy should have the same extension to distinguish them from the ectopic pregnancy codes.

15.6 HIV in a pregnant patient

During pregnancy, childbirth or the puerperium, a patient with HIV infection or an HIV-related illness should be assigned code O98.7, Human immunodeficiency [HIV] disease complicating pregnancy, childbirth and the puerperium, followed by the appropriate code(s) for the HIV disease. See guidelines 1.1.2 HIV in a pregnant patient.

15.7 Gestational diabetes

Codes for gestational (pregnancy-induced) diabetes are in subcategory O24.4. No other code from category O24, Diabetes mellitus in pregnancy, childbirth, and the puerperium, should be used with a code from O24.4. If a patient with gestational diabetes is treated with both diet and insulin, the default is for insulin-controlled.

15.8 Pre-existing conditions versus conditions due to the pregnancy

Certain categories in Chapter 15 distinguish between conditions of the mother that existed prior to pregnancy and those that are a direct result of pregnancy. When assigning codes from Chapter 15, it is important to assess if a condition was pre-existing prior to pregnancy or developed during or due to the pregnancy in order to assign the correct code.

Category O09, Supervision of high-risk pregnancy, includes codes for patients who have had complications with pregnancy in the past. Codes from this category may be used with other codes from Chapter 15.

O10, Pre-existing hypertension complicating pregnancy, childbirth and the puerperium, and O11, Pre-existing hypertensive disorder with superimposed proteinuria, are for cases when a pregnant woman has hypertension prior to pregnancy. Categories O12, Gestational [pregnancy-induced] edema and proteinuria without hypertension, O13, Gestational [pregnancy-induced] hypertension without significant proteinuria, and O14, Gestational [pregnancy-induced] hypertension with significant proteinuria, are for pregnancy-related conditions. Similarly, there are codes for pre-existing diabetes mellitus complicating pregnancy, O24.0-O24.3, and O24.8 and for gestational diabetes, O24.4.

Category O94, Maternal malignant neoplasm, traumatic injuries and abuse classified elsewhere but complicating pregnancy, childbirth and the puerperium, may be used for conditions that are pre-existing but will most often be used for cases when a malignancy is diagnosed or an injury occurs during pregnancy (See guideline 19.3.4.2 for instructions on coding of abuse in pregnancy). Categories O98, Maternal infectious and parasitic diseases classifiable elsewhere but complicating pregnancy, childbirth and the puerperium, and O99, Other maternal diseases classifiable elsewhere but complicating pregnancy, childbirth and the puerperium, will most often be assigned for pre-existing conditions, but may be used for conditions diagnosed during pregnancy. Subcategory O99.0, Anemia complicating pregnancy, childbirth and the puerperium, is only for use for pre-existing anemia. Postpartum anemia is coded O90.81. Anemia following delivery is very common in women who were not anemic before or during pregnancy due to the blood loss associated with delivery.

Pregnancy associated cardiomyopathy (O09.3) is unique in that it may be diagnosed in the third trimester of pregnancy but may continue to progress months after delivery. For this reason, it is referred to as peripartum cardiomyopathy. Mortality from this complication is very high. Heart transplantation may be the only treatment option. Code O09.3 is only for use when the cardiomyopathy develops as a result of pregnancy in a woman who did not have pre-existing heart disease.

Categories that do not distinguish between pre-existing and pregnancy-related conditions may be used for either. It is acceptable to use codes specifically for the puerperium with codes complicating pregnancy and childbirth if a condition arises postpartum during the delivery encounter.

15.9 Maternal care for fetal conditions
Categories O35, Maternal care for known or suspected fetal abnormality and damage, and O36, Maternal care for other fetal problems, are for problems with the fetus that affect the management of the pregnancy. Codes from these categories may be used for suspected problems with the fetus that have not been confirmed, as it is often not possible to confirm a fetal abnormality in utero.

15.10 Fetal care
Category O37, Fetal care for fetal abnormality and damage, is for use if treatment, such as a surgical procedure, is done to the fetus itself, in utero, or for complications of such treatment. Codes from this category are for use on the maternal record, or, on a fetal record, if an institution creates a unique record for the fetus. Category O37 is not for use on the record of a newborn.

Codes from Chapter 16, Certain conditions originating in the newborn (perinatal) period, are not for use on a mother's record. Perinatal codes are only for use on a newborn or infant record. They are not to be assigned to describe abnormalities of a fetus.

15.11 Outcome of delivery
A code from category Z37, Outcome of delivery, should be included on every maternal record when a delivery has occurred to indicate the status of the baby/babies born. These codes are not to be used on subsequent maternal records or on the newborn record.

15.12 Intrauterine death versus stillbirth
An intrauterine death is assigned either code O02.1, Missed abortion, for early fetal deaths before 20 weeks of gestation, or O36.4, Maternal care for intrauterine death, for late fetal deaths after 20 weeks of gestation. These codes are for use on the mother's record.

P95, Stillbirth, is only for use on a record designated for the baby. P95 is never for use on a maternal record.

A stillbirth code from category Z37, Outcome of delivery, is only for use on the record of a mother's delivery encounter, to indicate the status of the baby born. It is not for use with code P95.

15.13 Encounter for full-term uncomplicated delivery
Code O80, Encounter for full-term uncomplicated delivery, is for use in cases when a woman is admitted for a full-term normal delivery and delivers a single, healthy infant without any complications antepartum, during the delivery, or postpartum during the delivery episode.

Code O80 may be used if the patient had a complication at some point during her pregnancy but the complication is not present at the time of the admission for delivery.

Code O80 is always a principal diagnosis. It is not to be used if any other code from chapter 15 is needed to describe a current complication of the antenatal, delivery, or perinatal period. Additional codes from other chapters may be used with code O80 if they are not related to or are in any way complicating the pregnancy.

Z37.0, Single live birth, is the only outcome of delivery code appropriate for use with O80.

15.14 Encounter for cesarean delivery without indication
O82, Encounter for cesarean delivery without indication, is only for use for a delivery episode when a woman elects to have a cesarean delivery without medical need. It is not for use with any other code from Chapter 15 that would justify a cesarean delivery. It is always a principal diagnosis. It is a reason for encounter code. A procedure code for the cesarean delivery must accompany O82.

Z37.0, Single live birth, is the only outcome of delivery code appropriate for use with O82.

15.15 Routine prenatal visits
For routine prenatal visits when no complications are present, a code from category Z34, Encounter for supervision of normal pregnancy, should be used as the first-listed diagnosis. Codes from Z34 should not be used with Chapter 15 codes.

15.16 Encounter for termination of pregnancy
A woman being seen for an elective termination of an uncomplicated intrauterine pregnancy should be assigned Z33.2, Encounter for elective termination of pregnancy, as the first listed code.

Any immediate or subsequent complications of the procedure are identified with codes from categories O04, Complications following (induced) termination of pregnancy, or O07, Failed attempted termination of pregnancy.

Should a woman undergo a termination of a pregnancy due to fetal demise, other complications with the fetus or the health of the woman, the complication code(s) from Chapter 15 should be used, not code Z33.2. The termination is indicated with a procedure code.

15.17 The postpartum period
The postpartum period begins immediately after delivery and continues for six weeks following delivery.

A postpartum complication is any complication occurring within the six-week postpartum period.

Chapter 15 codes may also be used to describe pregnancy-related complications after the six-week period, if the physician documents that a condition is pregnancy related.

When a woman delivers outside the hospital prior to admission, and is admitted for routine postpartum care and no complications are noted, code Z39.0, Encounter for care and examination immediately after delivery, should be assigned as the first diagnosis. Should complications be noted, such as lacerations, the appropriate code for the complication from Chapter 15 should be assigned, not code Z39.0.

A delivery diagnosis code should not be used for a woman who has delivered prior to admission to the hospital. No outcome of delivery code should be used for these cases. Any postpartum procedures should be coded.

15.18 Sequelae of complication of pregnancy, childbirth, and the puerperium
Code O93, Sequelae of complication of pregnancy, childbirth, and the puerperium, is for use in those cases when an initial complication of a pregnancy develops a sequelae requiring care or treatment at a future date.

This code may be used at any time after the initial postpartum period.

Code O93 is sequenced following the code describing the sequelae of the complication.

15.19 Encounter for contraceptive and procreative management
Encounters for family planning and counseling, category Z30, Encounter for contraceptive management, and category Z31, Encounter for procreative management, should be included on an obstetric record either during the pregnancy or in the postpartum period, if applicable.

Codes from these categories may also be used for non-pregnant patients who are being seen for family planning and fertility services.

15.20 Encounter for antenatal screening
Code Z36, Encounter for antenatal screening, is for use for routine antenatal screening in pregnant women. Like all screening codes, it is only for use for women in whom no fetal

abnormalities are suspected. It may be used as a reason for visit code, or, in conjunction with other codes from Chapter 15.

Separate procedure codes for any screenings done must also be used.

Chapter 16: Certain conditions originating in the newborn (perinatal) period

16.1 General Chapter 16 guidelines
The perinatal period is defined as birth through the 28th day following birth.

All clinically significant conditions noted on routine newborn examination should be coded, the most serious or the one requiring the most care sequenced first. A condition is clinically significant if it requires:
clinical evaluation; or
therapeutic treatment; or
diagnostic procedures; or
extended length of hospital stay; or
increased nursing care and/or monitoring; or
has implications for future health care needs.

What constitutes a clinically significant condition is the same for perinatal records as for all other records, with the addition of the final point regarding implications for future health care needs.

Codes in this chapter are only for use on the newborn or infant record, not on the maternal record. Codes from this chapter are only applicable for liveborn infants.

Should a condition originate in the perinatal period, and continue throughout the life of the child, the perinatal code should continue to be used regardless of the age of the patient.

In cases where a baby has a condition that may be either due to the birth process (e.g., P35-P39, Infections specific to the perinatal period) or community acquired, the default should be complication of birth and a code from Chapter 16 should be used.

16.2 Liveborn infant according to place of birth and type of delivery
When coding the birth of an infant, assign a code from category Z38, Liveborn according to place of birth and type of delivery. A code from this category is assigned as a principal/first listed diagnosis and assigned only once to a newborn at the time of birth.

If the newborn is transferred to another institution, a code from Z38 is not used at the receiving hospital.

16.3 Newborn (suspected to be) affected by maternal conditions

A newborn may be suspected of having a problem due to a condition of the mother. Tests and treatment may be initiated even if the newborn is not showing obvious signs or symptoms of a problem. Categories P00-P04, Newborn affected by maternal factors and by complications of pregnancy, labor and delivery, are for use in these cases. Codes from these categories are still acceptable for use if any testing or treatment is done, even if no problem with the infant is determined. Should a problem with the baby be confirmed, codes from Chapter 16 to identify the specific condition should be used, followed by a code from the P00-P04 series.

16.4 Congenital anomalies in a newborn

Assign the appropriate code(s) from Chapter 17, Congenital malformations, deformations and chromosomal abnormalities, as additional diagnoses when a specific abnormality is diagnosed for a newborn. See guideline 17.1 Coding of syndromes.

16.5 Prematurity and low birth weight

Codes from category P05, Disorders of newborn related to slow fetal growth and fetal malnutrition, and subcategories P07.0, Extremely low birth weight newborn, and P07.1, Other low birth weight newborn, specify birth weight. Codes from subcategories P07.2, Extreme immaturity of newborn, and P07.3, Other preterm newborn, specify weeks of gestation. For birth weight, select the code that corresponds to the first weight recorded for the newborn. For weeks of gestation, select the code for the number of completed weeks of gestation.

Both birth weight and gestational age are usually documented. Both should be coded, with birth weight sequenced before gestational age. These codes should be used along with all other appropriate codes for the complications of preterm birth or low birth weight. The low birth weight code will normally be the first code following the Z38 unless a particularly serious complication, such as an infection or hemorrhage, receives the primary focus of treatment.

16.6 Low birth weight and immaturity status

Codes from subcategory Z91.7, Low birth weight and immaturity status, are for use as personal status codes for a child or adult who was small as a newborn. See guideline 21.2.6 Status.

16.7 Newborn affected by intrauterine procedure

Code P96.5, Complication to newborn due to (fetal) intrauterine procedure, not elsewhere classified, is for use on the newborn record to indicate that a procedure done on the newborn when he/she was still in utero, caused a complication(s) that is still affecting the newborn. Additional code(s) should be used with P96.5 to identify the complication(s).

16.8 Stillbirth

Code P95, Stillbirth, is only for use for institutions that maintain separate records for stillbirths. No other code should be used with P95. Code P95 should not be used on the mother's record. A stillbirth code from category Z37, Outcome of delivery, is only for use on the record of a mother's delivery encounter to indicate the status of the baby born. It is not for use with code

P95.

Chapter 17: Congenital malformations, deformations and chromosomal abnormalities
Codes from Chapter 17 may be used for any patient, regardless of the patient's age. Many of the conditions from this chapter are life-long.

17.1 Coding of syndromes
Congenital anomalies or syndromes may occur as a set of symptoms or multiple malformations. If the syndrome does not have a specific code, a code should be assigned for each presenting manifestation of the syndrome, from any chapter in the classification. For syndromes with specific codes, additional codes may be assigned to identify manifestations not included in the specific code.

Chapter 18: Symptoms, signs and abnormal clinical and laboratory findings, not elsewhere classified

18.1 General Chapter 18 guidelines
Codes from Chapter 18 are for use to describe the signs and symptoms that are bringing the patient in for care, and as final diagnoses when no definitive condition has been established at the end of an encounter.

A symptom code should be used with a confirmed diagnosis if the symptom is not always associated with that diagnosis, such as the use various signs and symptom associated with complex syndromes.

Many codes within other chapters of the ICD-10-CM are combination codes that include the diagnosis and the most common symptoms of that diagnosis. When using a combination code, a secondary code for the associated symptom is not necessary.

18.2 Severe sepsis and septic shock
Severe sepsis is defined as sepsis accompanied by associated organ dysfunction in one or more organs. Severe sepsis may result from serious insult to the body such as burns or other trauma that precipitates infection. Septic shock may occur with severe sepsis

A minimum of three codes are required to fully code a case of severe sepsis. The first code should be the infection code, usually a code from Chapter 1. The second code required is a code from subcategory R65.2, Severe sepsis. The codes under R65.2 indicate if septic shock is present. The third code(s) assigned identifies any associated organ dysfunction. A use additional code note with a list of commonly associated organ dysfunction codes is provided under R65.2.

See guideline 1.2 Sepsis.

18.3 Encounter for pain management

The reason for visit for a patient with a serious, chronic health problem or who has undergone complex treatments may be pain management. In such a case, the pain code should be the first listed or principal diagnosis. Category R52, Pain, not elsewhere classified, has subcategories for acute pain (R52.0-), chronic intractable pain (R52.1-), and other chronic pain (R52.2-). Within each subcategory are specified codes for postoperative pain and pain in neoplastic disease, as well as unspecified pain. Generally, patients admitted for pain management suffer from chronic intractable pain. Patients who have serious postoperative pain may also be admitted for pain management.

The underlying condition causing the pain should also be coded, but it should not be the first listed if the reason for the encounter and the treatment given is for pain management. Codes from R52 may also be used as secondary codes if pain management is a component of treatment for another health problem.

Category R52 is not for use in place of site-specific pain codes. The site-specific pain codes are for use to describe the symptom that leads a physician to perform a diagnostic work-up.

18.4 Falling

Code R26.81, Falling, should not be confused with the external cause codes for falls. The external cause fall codes describe the event that causes an injury. Code R26.81 is the code to be assigned when a patient tends to fall when attempting to walk.

R26.81 may be used in conjunction with an external cause code for falls, if the patient sustains an injury due to a fall. The external cause code describes the type of fall. The injury code should be the first listed code. The underlying condition that is responsible for the patient's tendency to fall should be coded first, if known.

18.5 Glasgow coma scale

ICD-10-CM contains the Glasgow coma scale (R40.2-) to be used in conjunction with traumatic brain injury codes or sequelae of cerebrovascular accident codes. Three codes, one from each subcategory, are needed to complete the scale.

If multiple coma assessments are done, a patient should receive an initial scale rating at time of admission and a final rating at discharge. Each facility needs to establish an in-house policy to determine which scale rating(s) to record on the medical record. An extension must be added to the coma codes to indicate which rating(s) is being maintained for the final record.

18.6 Death NOS

Code R99, Ill-defined and unknown cause of mortality, is only for use in the very limited circumstance when a patient who has already died is brought into the emergency department or other healthcare facility and is pronounced dead upon arrival. It does not represent the discharge disposition of death.

Chapter 19: Injury, poisoning and certain other consequences of external causes

Chapter 19 is divided into two sections, the "S" codes and the "T" codes. The "S" codes are the traumatic injury codes. The "T" codes are the burns and corrosions, poisonings and toxic effects, adverse effects and underdosing, complications of medical care and other such consequences of external causes.

19.1 Chapter 19 code extensions

Most categories in Chapter 19 have 7th character extensions that are required for each applicable code. There are three extensions used for most categories: a, initial encounter, d, subsequent encounter, and q, sequela. Fracture categories have different extensions. See guideline 19.2.2.1 Fracture extensions.

19.1.1 Extensions "a" and "d"

Extension a, initial encounter, is for use only for the initial (first) encounter for treatment of an injury. All subsequent encounters require extension d, subsequent encounter. An injury code with extension "d" may be used for as long as a patient is receiving treatment for an injury. The use of the extensions will enable the tracking of injury treatment for the entire course of treatment while still identifying the type of injury. See guideline 21.2.9, Aftercare.

If an injury is not new at the time of the first encounter, due to the patient's delay in seeking treatment, it is still considered the initial encounter. However, even if a physician is seeing a patient for treatment of an injury for the first time, if treatment for the injury has been provided by any other medical professional previously, it should be coded as a subsequent treatment encounter. The default extension, in cases when it is not known, is extension a, initial treatment.

19.1.2 Extension "q"

Extension q, sequela, is for use for complications or conditions that arise as a direct result of an injury, such as scar formation after a burn. The scars are sequelae of the burn. When using extension "q," it is necessary to use both the injury code that precipitated the sequela and the code for the sequela itself. The "q" is added only to the injury code, not the code that specifies the sequela. The "q" identifies the injury responsible for the sequela. The sequela is sequenced first, followed by the injury code.

19.2 "S" codes

The injury codes are very specific, but provide a great deal of detail. Each injury code describes a single component of an injury. Assign a separate code for each component of an injury. As many codes as are needed to fully describe the injury should be used. At each category, there are instructional notes that indicate which other codes may be required to fully describe an injury. For example, at all open wound categories there is an instructional note to code any associated wound infection.

When sequencing injury codes, the most severe injury should be sequenced first.

A wound code from this chapter should not be used for normal, healing surgical wounds.

The "S" codes are divided into body sections, head (S00-S09), neck (S10-S19), thorax (S20-S29), abdomen, lower back, lumbar spine and pelvis (S30-S39), shoulder and upper arm (S40-S49), elbow and forearm (S50-S59), wrist and hand (S60-S69), hip and thigh (S70-S79), knee and lower leg (S80-S89), and ankle and foot (S90-S99).

Within each body section are categories for types of injuries: superficial wounds, open wounds, fractures, dislocations, injuries to nerves, injuries to blood vessels, crush injuries and injuries to the internal organs that are specific to the body section.

19.2.1 Superficial and open wounds
Superficial wounds are divided into: contusions, abrasions, blisters, external constriction (such as, a rubber band constricting a finger), superficial foreign body, insect bite and other superficial bite.

Open wounds are divided into: lacerations without foreign body, laceration with foreign body, puncture wound without foreign body, puncture wound with foreign body, and open bite.

There may be overlap or imprecision in describing these types of wounds in medical record documentation. It is necessary to assign codes based on the terms used in the record. If a wound is described as a laceration, it is coded to laceration. If it is described as an abrasion, it is coded to abrasion. Bite NOS defaults to open bite.

Superficial wounds are not coded when associated with more severe injuries of the same site.

19.2.2 Fractures
Fractures are coded individually by site. As many fracture codes as are needed to fully describe the fractures should be used. The most serious fracture is sequenced first. A fracture not indicated as open or closed should be coded to closed. A fracture not indicated whether displaced or not displaced should be coded to displaced.

19.2.2.1 Fracture extensions
In addition to the extensions for initial encounter, subsequent encounter and sequela that the other "S" codes have, the fracture codes have additional extensions indicating open or closed fracture, routine healing, delayed healing, nonunion and malunion of fractures.

Open fractures of long bones have extensions for degree of severity. The default extension for open fractures is b, initial encounter for treatment of open fracture type I or II.

The fracture extensions are unique to each type of bone and type of fracture. It is necessary to review the fracture extensions carefully before assigning an extension.

A fracture code with the appropriate extension should be assigned for as long as a patient is receiving treatment for a fracture. The extension may change with each encounter.

19.2.3 Crush injuries
The crush injury code should be sequenced first, followed by all applicable codes that indicate the specific injuries associated with the crushing.

19.2.4 Amputations
Amputation codes include the fracture of the bone of the amputated site. No additional fracture code is necessary with an amputation code. If not documented whether complete or partial, an amputation should be coded to complete.

19.2.5 Spinal cord injuries
For each section of spinal cord injury, the code for the highest level of injury for that section of the cord should be used. So, for example, for injuries of the cervical spinal cord, code to the highest level of injury of the cervical cord if the cervical cord is injured in more than one location. If a patient has a cord injury at more than one section of the cord, cervical and thoracic, for instance, use a code for the highest level of injury for each section. If the patient has a complete lesion of the cord, it is not necessary to use any additional codes for spinal cord injuries below the level of the complete lesion.

19.2.6 Use of an external cause code (Chapter 20) with an injury code
When an injury code is assigned to a medical record, a corresponding external cause code must also be assigned to identify the cause of the injury. Additionally, an activity code (Y93) and a place of occurrence code (Y92) should also be assigned. Place of occurrence codes are not required for adverse effects, poisonings and toxic effects.

Should an injury be work related (activity done for income), assign an activity code with extension 2.

See guidelines for Chapter 20 for instructions on the use of external cause codes.

19.3 "T" codes

19.3.1 Burns and corrosions
The ICD-10-CM distinguishes between burns and corrosions. The burn codes are for thermal burns, except sunburns, that come from a heat source, such as a fire or hot appliance. The burn codes are also for burns resulting from electricity and radiation. Corrosions are burns due to chemicals. If a burn is a thermal burn, a burn code should be used. If a burn is a chemical burn, a corrosion code should be used. The guidelines for burns and corrosions are the same.

Current burns and corrosions of the external body surface (T20-T25) are classified by site and by depth: first degree (erythema), second degree (blistering), and third degree (full-thickness involvement). Burns of the eye and internal organs (T26-T28) are classified by site, but not by degree.

Assign separate codes for each burn or corrosion site. Sequence first the code that reflects the highest degree of burn or corrosion when more than one site is affected. Sequence internal burns and corrosions before burns of the external body surface if they are more severe or require more extensive treatment. Classify burns or corrosions of the same local site, but of different degrees, to the highest degree recorded in the diagnosis.

19.3.1.1 Non-healing or infected burns and corrosions
Non-healing burns or corrosions are coded as acute burns or corrosions. Necrosis of burned skin should be coded as a non-healed burn.

For any documented infected burn site, use an additional code for the infection.

19.3.1.2 Burn NOS, Corrosion NOS
Code T30.0, Burn of unspecified body region, unspecified degree, and code T30.4, Corrosion of unspecified body region, unspecified degree, should only be used if the location of the burns or corrosions are not documented. These codes are never for use in the inpatient setting.

19.3.1.3 Burns and corrosions classified according to extent of body surface involved
Assign an additional code from category T31, Burns classified according to extent of body surface involved, or T32, Corrosions classified according to extent of body surface involved, to indicate the total body surface burned. It is advisable to use these codes to provide data for evaluating burn morbidity and mortality, such as that needed by burn units. It is also recommended to use a code from category T31 for reporting purposes when there is mention of a third-degree burn involving 20 percent or more of the body surface.

Categories T31 and T32 are based on the classic "rule of nines" in estimating body surface involved: head and neck are assigned nine percent, each arm nine percent, each leg 18 percent, the anterior trunk 18 percent, posterior trunk 18 percent, and genitalia one percent. Physicians may change these percentage assignments where necessary to accommodate infants and children who have proportionately larger heads than adults and patients who have large buttocks, thighs, or abdomen that involve burns or corrosions.

19.3.1.4 Use of an external cause code with burns and corrosions
External cause code(s) should be used with burns and corrosions to indicate the source of the burn, the place where it occurred and the activity of the patient at the time of the incident.

19.3.1.5 Sequela of burns and corrosions
Extension "q" should be assigned to a burn or corrosion code to indicate that a sequela of the burn or corrosion exists. See guideline 19.1.2 Extension q.

When appropriate, both a code for a current burn or corrosion with extension "a" or "d", and a burn or corrosion code with extension "q" may be assigned on the same record. Burns and corrosions do not heal at the same rate and a current healing wound may still exist with a sequela of a healed burn or corrosion.

19.3.2 Poisonings, toxic effects, adverse effects and underdosing
A poisoning is an overdose of a drug or a drug given or taken in error. When an error is made in a drug prescription or in the administration of a drug by a physician, nurse, patient, or other person, it is considered a poisoning. If a nonprescribed drug or medicinal agent is taken in combination with a correctly prescribed and properly administered drug, any drug toxicity or other reaction resulting from the interaction of the two drugs is classified as a poisoning.

A toxic effect is a poisoning due to a toxic substance that has no medicinal use.

An adverse effect is a reaction to a drug that is taken as prescribed and is properly administered.

Underdosing is taking less of a medication than is prescribed by a physician or the manufacturer's instruction with a resulting negative health consequence. A noncompliance (Z91.12-, Z91.13-) or failure in dosage during surgical or medical care (Y63.-) code must be used with an underdosing code to indicate intent.

Categories T36-T50, Poisoning, adverse effects and underdosing by drugs, medicaments and biological substances, and T51-T65, Toxic effects of substances chiefly nonmedicinal as to source, are the categories for the different classes of drugs and chemical agents that may cause a poisoning, toxic effect or adverse effect.

Poisonings and toxic effects have an associated intent: accidental, intentional self-harm, assault, and undetermined. The final characters 1,2, 3, and 4 for each code in these categories, usually the 6th character, indicates the intent. The final character 5 for categories T36-T50 indicates an adverse effect. The final character 6 for categories T36-T50 indicate underdosing.
The final characters are as follows:
1   accidental (unintentional)
2   intentional self-harm
3   assault
4   undetermined
5   adverse effect (for categories T36-T50 only)
6   underdosing (for categories T36-T50 only)

When no intent is indicated, the default is accidental. Undetermined intent is only for use when there is specific documentation in the medical record that the intent of the poisoning or toxic effect cannot be determined.

No additional external cause code is required for poisonings, toxic effects, adverse effects and underdosing codes.

19.3.2.1 5th character "x" place holder
The 5th character "x" at many of the codes in categories T36-T65 is a dummy place holder to allow for possible future expansion. The "x" must remain in the code and no other character should be used in its place.

19.3.2.2 Sequencing of poisonings, toxic effects, adverse effects and underdosing
A code from categories T36-T65 is sequenced first, followed by the code(s) that specifies the nature of the poisoning, toxic effect or adverse effect.

19.3.2.3 Poisonings, toxic effects, adverse effects and underdosing in a pregnant patient
Codes from Chapter 15, Pregnancy, childbirth, and the puerperium, are always sequenced first on a medical record. A code from subcategory O94.2, Injury, poisoning and certain other consequences of external causes complicating pregnancy, childbirth, and the puerperium, should be sequenced first, followed by the appropriate poisoning, toxic effect, adverse effect or underdosing code and the additional code(s) that specify the nature of the poisoning, toxic effect, adverse effect or underdosing.

19.3.3 Other "T" codes that include the external cause
In addition to the poisonings, toxic effects, adverse effects and underdosing, certain other "T" codes are combination codes that include the external cause. For example, the codes in categories T17-T19, Effects of foreign body entering through natural orifice, identifies both the foreign body, as well as the resulting injury. The intent for these codes is accidental. No secondary external cause code is needed.

For category T71, Asphyxiation, in addition to the external cause and the resulting injury, the intent is included at the final character. The intent codes are the same as those for the poisonings, toxic effects and adverse effects codes.

The final characters are as follows:

1   accidental (unintentional)
2   intentional self-harm
3   assault
4   undetermined

When no intent is indicated, the default is accidental. Undetermined intent is only for use when there is specific documentation in the medical record that the intent of the poisoning or toxic effect cannot be determined.

19.3.4 Adult and child abuse, neglect and other maltreatment

The ICD-10-CM has two categories for abuse and neglect, T74, Adult and child abuse, neglect and other maltreatment, confirmed, and T76, Adult and child abuse, neglect and other maltreatment, suspected. A code from these categories is sequenced first, followed by any accompanying mental health or injury code(s).

If the documentation in the medical record states abuse or neglect it is coded to confirmed. It is coded as suspected if it is documented as suspected.

If a suspected case of abuse, neglect or mistreatment is ruled out during an encounter, code Z04.71, Suspected adult physical and sexual abuse, ruled out, or code Z04.72, Suspected child physical and sexual abuse, ruled out, should be used, not a code from T76.

19.3.4.1 Use of an external cause code with an abuse or neglect code

For cases of confirmed physical abuse, an external cause code from the assault section (X92-Y08) should be added to identify the cause of any physical injuries. A perpetrator code (Y07) should be added when the perpetrator of the abuse is known.

19.3.4.2 Abuse and other maltreatment in a pregnant patient

Codes from Chapter 15, Pregnancy, childbirth, and the puerperium, are always sequenced first on a medical record. A code(s) from subcategories O94.3, Physical abuse complicating pregnancy, childbirth, and the puerperium, O94.4, Sexual abuse complicating pregnancy, childbirth, and the puerperium, and O94.5, Psychological abuse complicating pregnancy, childbirth, and the puerperium, should be sequenced first, followed by any accompanying mental health or injury code(s). No code from category T74 or T76 is needed.

19.3.5 Complications of surgical and medical care, not elsewhere classified

19.3.5.1 Complication codes that include the external cause
As with certain other T codes, some of the "complications of care" codes have the external cause included in the code. An example is subcategory T81.5, Complications of foreign body accidentally left in body following procedure. The code includes the nature of the complication as well as the type of procedure that caused the complication. No external cause code indicating the type of procedure is necessary with a code from T81.5.

19.3.5.2 Mechanical complications
A mechanical complication of a medical device, implant or graft is defined as one of the following:
    Mechanical breakdown
    Displacement or malposition
    Leakage
    Obstruction
    Perforation
    Protrusion

If a repair of a medical device, implant or graft is done to correct one of the complications defined above, a mehancial complication code should be assigned.

19.3.5.3 Organ Transplant complications
Organ transplant rejection, failure or infection are complications. Category T86, Complications of transplanted organs and tissue, has codes for these specified types of complications. Should a physician document that another problem a patient may be experiencing is associated with a transplanted organ, it should also be coded as a complication. See guideline 21.2.6 Status, for transplant status coding.

19.3.5.4 Complications of care codes within the body system chapters
Intraoperative and postprocedural complication codes are found within the body system chapters with codes specific to the organs and structures of that body system. These codes should be sequenced first, followed by a code(s) for the specific complication, if applicable.

The categories are as follows:
D78   Intraoperative and postprocedural complications of procedures on the spleen
E36   Intraoperative and postprocedural complications of endocrine procedures
G97   Intraoperative and postprocedural complications and disorders of nervous system, not elsewhere classified
H59   Intraoperative and postprocedural complications and disorders of eye and adnexa, not elsewhere classified
H95   Intraoperative and postprocedural complications and disorders of ear and mastoid process, not elsewhere classified

I97 Intraoperative and postprocedural complications and disorders of the circulatory system, not elsewhere classified

J95 Intraoperative and postprocedural complications and disorders of the respiratory system, not elsewhere classified

K91 Intraoperative and postprocedural complications and disorders of the digestive system, not elsewhere classified

L76 Intraoperative and postprocedural complications of dermatologic procedures

M96 Intraoperative and postprocedural complications and disorders of the musculoskeletal system, not elsewhere classified

N99 Intraoperative complications and postprocedural disorders of genitourinary system, not elsewhere classified

Chapter 20: External causes of morbidity

<u>20.1 General Chapter 20 guidelines</u>

External cause codes for injuries and other health conditions provide data for research and prevention strategies. These codes capture the cause of the injury or health condition, the intent (unintentional (accidental), intentional self-harm, or, assault), the place where the event occurred, and the activity of the patient at the time of the event. **External cause codes are never to be recorded as a principal/first listed diagnosis**.

An external cause code may be used with any code in the classification that is a health condition due to an external cause. Though they are most applicable to injuries, they are also valid for use with such things as infections or diseases due to an external source, and other health conditions, such as a heart attack, that occurs during strenuous physical activity. They are for use in any health care setting.

Assign as many external cause codes as necessary to fully explain each cause. The sequencing of multiple external cause codes is based on the sequence of events leading to the injury. If only one external cause code can be recorded, assign the external cause code that relates to the principal/first-listed diagnosis. The place of occurrence and activity code are sequenced after the main external cause code. Regardless of the number of external cause codes assigned there should be only one place of occurrence code and one activity code assigned to a record.

Certain of the external cause codes are combination codes that identify sequential events that result in an injury, such as a fall that results in striking against an object. The injury may be due to either event or both. The combination external cause code used should correspond to the sequence of events regardless of which caused the most serious injury.

External cause codes for child and adult abuse take sequencing priority over all other external cause codes. See guideline 19.3.4, Adult and child abuse, neglect and other maltreatment.

External cause codes for terrorism take sequencing priority over all other external cause codes except child and adult abuse.

External codes for cataclysmic events take sequencing priority over all other external cause codes except child and adult abuse and terrorism.

External cause codes for transport accidents take sequencing priority over all other external cause codes except cataclysmic events, child and adult abuse and terrorism.

The selection of the appropriate external cause code is guided by the Index to External Causes, a separate index in the ICD-10-CM, and by the instructional notes in Chapter 20. The main term for the external cause is located in the index. The code indicated in the index for the main term is verified in the Tabular List of Chapter 20. The conventions and rules for the classification also apply to Chapter 20. See guidelines Section I, ICD-10-CM Conventions, and Section II, General

Coding Guidelines.

The external cause codes are divided into sections. The first section, V00-X58, are the unintentional (accidental) injuries. The second section, X71-X83, are the intentional self-harm categories. The third section, X92-Y08, are the categories for assault. Categories Y21-Y33 are for undetermined intent. There are substantially more unintentional categories due to the nature of external cause codes. For prevention purposes, it is important to capture data on the cause of unintentional injuries. For self-harm and assault, it is the intent itself that is most important to capture.

There are also sections for legal interventions, operations of war, military operations, terrorism, complications of medical and surgical care and supplemental factors related to causes of morbidity classified elsewhere. Categories for place of occurrence and activity are located in the final section.

The external cause categories include:
Unintentional (accidental) injuries
    Transport accidents
    Falls
    Struck by or caught between objects
    Contact with objects
    Firearms
    Explosions
    Exposure to animate and inanimate mechanical forces and other external causes
    Non-transport drowning and submersion
    Smoke, fire and flames
    Cataclysms and other forces of nature
Intentional self-harm
Assaults
Undetermined intent
Legal interventions
Operations of war/ Military operations
Terrorism
Complications of medical and surgical care
Place of occurrence
Activity code
Other supplemental factors related to causes of morbidity classified elsewhere

Poisonings, toxic effects, adverse effects and underdosing and their associated intent are located in Chapter 19, categories T36-T65. See guideline 19.3.2 Poisonings, toxic effects, adverse effects, and underdosing.

No external cause code from Chapter 20 is needed if the external cause and intent is included in a code from another chapter.

20.2 External cause code extensions

Codes from categories V00-Y35 require an extension to indicate whether the encounter is the initial encounter for treatment, a subsequent encounter for treatment, or the sequelae of an event. The extensions for these categories are as follows:

a initial encounter

d subsequent encounter

q sequelae

These extensions match the extensions for the non-fracture T codes that have extensions.

An external cause code may be used for every health care encounter for the duration of treatment of an illness or injury. Extension "a" should be used for the initial encounter, "d" for every subsequent encounter, and "q" for any encounter for treatment of the sequelae of an external cause. The initial encounter is the first time a patient is seen by any health care provider in any setting for treatment of an injury. It is still considered the initial encounter even if the injury was sustained earlier and the patient delayed seeking treatment. Any encounter after the initial encounter is recorded as subsequent treatment.

Different extensions are needed for Y93, Activity code. See guideline 20.10 Activity code.

No extensions are required for categories Y62-Y84, Complications of medical and surgical care, Y90, Evidence of alcohol involvement determined by blood alcohol level, Y92, Place of occurrence, (See guideline 20.9 Place of occurrence), or Y95, Nosocomial condition.

20.3 Unintentional (accidental) injuries:

The default for external cause is unintentional. If there is no documentation in the medical record as to the intent of an injury, it should be assigned an "unintentional intent" external cause code.

The external cause categories V00-X58 are "unintentional intent" categories.

20.3.1 Transport accidents

See the Tabular list at V00-V99 for definitions related to transport accidents. It is important to review all instructional notes at the transport accident categories to properly select the correct code.

This section is structured in 12 groups reflecting the victim's mode of transportation. The type of vehicle the victim is an occupant in is identified in the first two characters since it is seen as the most important factor to identify for prevention purposes.

A transport accident is one in which the vehicle involved must be moving or running or in use for transport purposes at the time of the accident.

When accidents involving more than one kind of transport are recorded, the following order of precedence should be used:
aircraft and spacecraft (V95-V97)
watercraft (V90-V94)
other modes of transport (V00-V89, V98-V99)

Where transport accident descriptions do not specify the victim as being a vehicle occupant and the victim is described by terms such as, crushed, dragged, hit, run over etc., classify the victim as a pedestrian.

If no documentation is available as to whether the victim was the driver or occupant of a vehicle, classify the victim as an occupant.

Use additional external cause codes with a transport accident code to identify:
the use of a cell phone or other electronic equipment contributing to the accident (Y93.5-)
whether an airbag contributed to any injury (W22.1)
the type of street or road where the accident occurred, if known, (Y92.4-)

20.3.2 Falls

Categories W00-W19, Falls, include the main fall codes in Chapter 20. These codes are for standard types of falls, such as, due to ice and snow, falling from stairs or off a ladder. There are other fall codes in Chapter 20 for falls associated with other causes, such as, fires, watercraft accidents, pedestrian conveyance accidents or with subsequent striking against objects. A complete review of the index is necessary when selecting a fall code to be sure that the correct category and code are assigned.

20.4 Assault

If a patient's injury has been intentionally inflicted by another person, by any means, with intent to kill or injure, it is classified as an assault. A code from the assault categories (X92-Y08), should be used to record the external cause of the injury.

Assault does not include injuries as a result of legal intervention, operations of war, military operations or terrorism. See guidelines 20.5 Undetermined intent, and 20.6 Legal interventions, 20.7, Operations of war/military operations, and 20.8 Terrorism.

20.4.1 Adult and child abuse, neglect and maltreatment

The external cause for adult and child abuse is classified as assault. Any of the assault codes may be used to indicate the external cause of any injury resulting from abuse. For confirmed cases of abuse, neglect and maltreatment, when the perpetrator is known, a code from Y07, Perpetrator of maltreatment and neglect, should accompany any other assault codes. See guideline 19.3.4 Adult and child abuse, neglect and maltreatment.

20.5 Undetermined intent
The default for injuries when the documentation does not indicate intent is unintentional. Codes from categories Y20-Y33, Events of undetermined intent, are only for use when the documentation in the record specifically states that the intent cannot be determined.

20.6 Legal interventions
The codes from category Y35, Legal intervention, are for use for any injury documented as sustained as a result of an encounter with any law enforcement official, serving in any capacity at the time of the encounter, whether on-duty or off-duty. The sixth-character for the legal intervention codes identifies the victim, a law enforcement official, a bystander or the suspect of a crime

The extensions for Y35 are the same as for the majority of categories in Chapter 20:
a   initial encounter
d   subsequent encounter
q   sequelae

See guideline 20.2 External cause code extensions.

20.7 Operations of war/ Military operations
Category Y36, Operations of war, is limited to classifying injuries sustained during a time of declared war and that are directly due to the war. Y37, Military operations, is for use to classify injuries to military and civilian personnel occurring during peacetime on military property or during routine military exercises or operations.

The extensions for Y36 and Y37 are the same as for the majority of categories in Chapter 20:
a   initial encounter
d   subsequent encounter
q   sequelae

Transport accidents during peacetime involving military vehicles that are off military property are included with the transport accidents, not in Y36 or Y37.

20.8 Terrorism
When the cause of an injury is identified by the Federal Bureau of Investigations (FBI) as terrorism, the first-listed external cause code should be a code from category Y38, Terrorism. The definition of terrorism is found at the beginning of the category. The code selected from Y38 should be the only external cause code assigned to a medical record. More than one Y38 code may be assigned if the injury is the result of more than one mechanism of terrorism.

Only injuries confirmed to be due to terrorism should be assigned a code from Y38. Suspected cases should be classified as assault.

Y38.9, Terrorism, secondary effects, is for use to identify injuries occurring subsequent to a terrorist attack, not due to the initial attack itself.

The extensions for Y38 are the same as for the majority of categories in Chapter 20:
a   initial encounter
d   subsequent encounter
q   sequelae

20.9 Place of Occurrence
Codes from category Y92, Place of occurrence of the external cause, are secondary codes for use with other external cause codes to identify the location of the patient at the time of injury. A place of occurrence code is used only once, at the initial encounter for treatment. Only one code from Y92 should be recorded on a medical record. A place of occurrence code should be used in conjunction with an activity code, Y93.

Use place of occurrence code Y92.9 if the place is not stated or is not applicable. Place of occurrence codes are not necessary with poisonings, toxic effects, adverse effects or underdosing codes.

No extensions are used for Y92.

20.10 Activity code
Codes from category Y93, Activity code, are secondary codes for use with other external cause codes to identify the activity of the patient at the time of the injury. An activity code is used only once, at the initial encounter for treatment. Only one code from Y93 should be recorded on a medical record. An activity code should be used in conjunction with a place of occurrence code, Y92.

Use activity code Y93.9 if the activity of the patient is not stated or is not applicable.

Specific 7th character extensions are required for Y93:
1   non-work related activity
2   work-related activity
3   student activity
4   military activity

If a patient is a student but is injured while performing an activity for income, use extension 2.

Chapter 21: Factors influencing health status and contact with health service

21.1 General Chapter 21 Guidelines

Chapter 21, Factors influencing health status and contact with health services, (the Z codes) are provided to deal with occasions when circumstances other than a disease or injury classifiable to the other chapters of the ICD-10-CM are recorded as a reason for encounters with a health care provider. There are 4 primary circumstances for the use of Z codes:

1. When a person who is not currently sick has a health care encounter for some specific reason, such as, to act as an organ donor, to receive prophylactic care, such as inoculations or health screenings, or to receive counseling on a health related issue.

2. When a person with a resolving disease or injury or a chronic, long-term condition requiring continuous care has a health care encounter for specific aftercare of that disease or injury, such as, dialysis for renal disease or chemotherapy for a malignancy. A diagnosis/symptom code, not a Z code, should be used whenever a current, acute condition is being treated or a sign or symptom is being studied.

3. When circumstances or problems influence a person's health status but are not in themselves a current illness or injury.

4. For newborns, to indicate birth status

Z codes are for use in both the inpatient and outpatient setting but are generally more applicable in the outpatient setting.

Z codes may be used as either principal/first-listed codes or as secondary codes, depending on the circumstances of the encounter. Certain Z codes may only be first-listed, others only secondary. The Z code Table at the end of the Z code guidelines identifies the sequencing restrictions for the Z code categories.

A Z code may be assigned based on any documentation in the medical record, including nursing and therapist notes, unless the Z code is the principal/first listed, in which case there must be physician documentation.

Z codes indicate a reason for an encounter. They are not procedure codes. A corresponding procedure code must accompany a Z code to describe a procedure performed.

21.2 The Z code categories

21.2.1 General and administrative examinations

The categories for general and administrative examinations describe encounters for routine examinations. These are "reason for visit" categories. Any procedures performed must be identified with separate procedure codes from the appropriate procedure classification. The codes from these categories are first listed codes. They are not for use if the examination is for diagnosis of a suspected condition or for treatment purposes. In such cases, a confirmed diagnosis, sign or symptom code should be used.

Category Z00, Encounter for general examination without complaint, suspected or reported diagnosis, and category Z01, Encounter for other special examination without complaint or suspected or reported diagnosis, include subcategories for general medical examinations, including eye, ear, and dental examinations, general laboratory and radiology examinations, routine child health examinations, as well as encounters for examinations for potential organ donors and controls for participants in clinical trials. Category Z02, Encounter for administrative examinations, includes codes for such things as pre-employment physicals.

The final character of the general health examination codes distinguishes between "without abnormal findings" and "with abnormal findings." For these encounters, if an abnormal condition is discovered, the code for "with abnormal findings" should be used. A secondary code for the specific abnormal finding should be used.

Subcategories Z00.02, Encounter for general laboratory examination, and Z00.03, Encounter for general radiology examination, are only for use if the only reason for the encounter is for routine blood work or x-rays that are a component of a general examination but are occurring independently of the full medical examination. They are not to be used if an encounter is for diagnostic lab work or x-rays. For such cases, codes for the sign or symptom or condition being investigated should be used.

Pre-operative examination codes, Z01.81-Z01.84, are for use only in those situations when a patient is being cleared for surgery and no other treatment is given.

Pre-existing and chronic conditions, as long as the examination does not focus on them, may also be assigned with codes from Z00-Z02.

21.2.2 Observation

An observation encounter is one when a person without a diagnosis is suspected of having an abnormal condition following an accident or incident, that might result in a health problem, but without signs or symptoms, that after examination and observation is ruled out. They are for use in very limited circumstances when a person is being observed for a suspected condition that is found not to exist. The fact that the patient may be scheduled for a return encounter following the initial observation encounter does not limit the use of an observation code.

There are two observation categories, Z03, Encounter for medical observation for suspected diseases and conditions, ruled out, and Z04, Encounter for observation for other reasons.

An observation code should not be used for a patient with any illness, injury or signs and symptoms. The illness, injury, signs or symptoms should be coded, with the corresponding external cause code. Pre-existing and chronic conditions may also be assigned with codes from Z03-Z04, as long as they are not associated with the suspected condition being observed.

21.2.3 Follow-up
The follow-up codes are for use to describe encounters for continuing surveillance following completed treatment of a disease, condition or injury. Follow-up infers that the condition has been fully treated and no longer exists. It should not be confused with aftercare that explain current treatment for a healing or long-term condition. See guideline 21.2.9 Aftercare.

Follow-up codes should be used in conjunction with history (of) codes to provide the full picture of the healed or treated condition. The follow-up code is sequenced first, followed by the history (of) code.

A follow-up code may be used for repeated visits, such as the long-term follow-up of cancer. If a condition is found to have recurred on a follow-up visit, the follow-up code should still be used, followed by the diagnosis code.

The two follow-up codes are Z08, Encounter for follow-up examination after completed treatment for malignant neoplasm, and Z09, Encounter for follow-up examination after completed treatment for conditions other than malignant neoplasm. When using Z08, it is necessary to assign the appropriate secondary code from category Z85, Personal history of primary and secondary malignant neoplasm.

21.2.4 Screening
Screening is the testing for disease or disease precursors in seemingly healthy individuals so that early detection and treatment can be provided for those who test positive for the disease. Screenings are recommended for many subgroups in a population, such as, a routine mammograms for women over 40, a fecal occult blood test or colonoscopy for anyone over 50, or an amniocentesis to rule out a fetal anomaly for pregnant women over 35, because the incidence of breast cancer and colon cancer in these subgroups is higher than in the general population, as is the incidence of Down syndrome in older mothers.

The testing of a person to rule out or confirm a suspected diagnosis because the patient has some sign or symptom is a diagnostic test, not a screening. For these cases, the code for the sign or symptom is used to explain the test, not the screening code.

A screening code may be a first listed code if the reason for the encounter is specifically the screening. They may also be used as an additional code(s) if the screening is done during an encounter for other health reasons. A screening code is not necessary if the screening is inherent to a routine examination, such as a pap smear done during a routine pelvic examination.

Should a condition be discovered during a screening, the screening code should still be used, followed by the code for the condition that is discovered.

The screening codes are "reason for visit" codes. A procedure code from the appropriate procedure classification is required to indicate which tests were performed.

The screening categories are:

Z11   Encounter for special screening examination for infectious and parasitic diseases
Z12   Encounter for special screening examination for malignant neoplasm
Z13   Encounter for special screening examination for other diseases and disorders

21.2.5 Contact/Exposure

Codes from Category Z20, Contact with and exposure to communicable diseases, are for patients who do not show any signs or symptoms of a disease but who have been exposed to it by close personal contact with an infected individual or are in an area where a disease is epidemic. These codes may be used as a first listed code to explain an encounter for testing, or, more commonly, as a secondary code to identify a potential risk.

21.2.6 Status

Status codes indicate that a patient is either a carrier of a disease or has the sequelae or residual of a past disease or condition. This includes such things as the use of a prosthetic or mechanical device. A status code is informative because the status may affect any current treatment and its outcome. A status code is distinct from a history code. A history code indicates that the patient no longer has a condition. See guideline 21.2.12 History (of).

The status Z categories/subcategories/codes are:

Z14   Genetic carrier
       This category indicates that a person is a carrier of a non-infectious condition that may be passed on genetically to any offspring. The carrier does not have the condition itself. Codes from Z14 are most often for use for pregnancy women who may pass on an hereditary condition to a fetus.
Z15   Genetic susceptibility to disease
       Codes from this category indicate that a person has a gene that increases the risk of getting certain conditions, most notably cancer. A code from Z15 will most often be for use to explain the reason for a prophylactic procedure.
Z16   Infection with drug-resistant microorganism
       This code indicates that a patient has an infection that is resistant to antibiotics. Sequence the infection code first.
Z21   Asymptomatic human immunodeficiency virus [HIV] infection status
       This code indicates that a patient has tested positive for HIV but has no signs or

symptoms of the disease. See guideline 1.1 Human immunodeficiency virus [HIV] disease.

Z22   Carrier of infectious disease

Carrier status indicates that a person harbors a specific organism of a disease without symptoms but is capable of transmitting the infection to others. This category is also for use for suspected carriers.

Z33.1 Pregnant state, incidental

This is a secondary code only for use when a pregnancy is in no way complicating the reason for a health care encounter. See guideline 15.1 General Chapter 15 Guidelines.

Z79   Long-term (current) drug therapy

This category indicates a patient's continuous use of a drug (prescribed or over the counter) for the long-term treatment of a condition or for prophylactic use. It does not indicate an addiction to a drug.

Z88   Allergy status to drugs, medicaments and biological substances

Drug allergies are life-long. Codes from this category should be added to a patient's record at every encounter to caution that a patient suffers from a drug allergy.

Z89   Acquired absence of limb

Z90   Acquired absence of organs, not elsewhere classified

Z91.0 Allergy status, other than to drugs and biological substances

This subcategory includes allergies to foods, insects, and other nonmedicinal substances, such as latex. Allergies are life-long. Codes from this subcategory should be added to a patient's record at every encounter to caution that a patient suffers from an allergy.

Z91.7 Low birth weight and immaturity status

Z93   Artificial opening status

Z94   Transplanted organ and tissue status

Z95   Presence of cardiac and vascular implants and grafts

Z96   Presence of other functional implants

Z97   Presence of other devices

Z98   Other postsurgical states

Z99   Dependence on enabling machines and devices, not elsewhere classified

Categories Z89-Z99 are for use only if there is no complication or malfunction of the organ or tissue replaced, of the amputation site, or the equipment on which the patient is dependent. These are always secondary codes.

21.2.7 Encounter for immunization/Immunization not carried out

Code Z23, Encounter for immunization, is for use to indicate that a patient is being seen to receive a prophylactic inoculation against a disease. **The injection itself must be indicated with a procedure code**. This code may be used as a secondary code if the inoculation is given as a part of preventive health care, such as a well-baby visit.

Immunizations against many communicable diseases is required in most states for admission to school or for employment. For persons who choose not to receive an immunization for personal or health reasons, a code from category Z28, Immunization not carried out, should be used to identify the reason a required immunization is not given.

21.2.8 Encounters for health services related to reproduction

The categories/code related to reproduction include:

Z30   Encounter for contraceptive management
Z31   Encounter for procreative management
Z32   Encounter for pregnancy test and instruction
Z33.2 Encounter for elective termination of pregnancy
       (Code Z33.1, Pregnancy state, incidental, is a status code)
Z34   Encounter for supervision of normal pregnancy
Z36   Encounter for antenatal screening
Z37   Outcome of delivery
Z38   Liveborn infant according to place of birth and type of delivery
Z39   Encounter for maternal postpartum care and examination

See guidelines for Chapter 15 for instructions on the use of codes from categories Z30-Z37, and code Z33.2.

See guidelines for Chapter 16 for instructions on the use of Z38.

These encounter codes identify the reason for visit. Any procedures performed must be identified with a procedure code from the appropriate procedure classification.

21.2.9 Aftercare

Aftercare visit codes, with such category titles as fitting and adjustment, and attention to artificial openings, cover situations when the initial treatment of a disease or injury has been performed and the patient requires continuing care during the healing or recovery phase, or for the long-term consequences of an illness. The aftercare Z codes should not be used if treatment is directed at a current disease or injury. The disease or injury code should be used in such cases. See guideline 19.1.1 Extensions "a" and "d".

The aftercare codes are generally first listed, "reason for visit" codes. An aftercare code may also be used as a secondary code, when some type of aftercare is provided in addition to another reason for an encounter and no diagnosis code is applicable. An example of this would be the closure of a colostomy during an encounter for treatment of another condition.

Certain aftercare codes need a secondary diagnosis code to describe the resolving condition or sequelae. For others, the condition is inherent in the code title.

Aftercare codes are not for use for mechanical complications or malfunctioning of a device. See guideline 19.3.5.2 Mechanical complications.

The aftercare categories are:

Z43   Encounter for attention to artificial openings
Z44   Encounter for fitting and adjustment of external prosthetic device
Z45   Encounter for adjustment and management of implanted device
Z46   Encounter for fitting and adjustment of other devices
Z47   Orthopedic aftercare
Z48   Encounter for other surgical aftercare
Z49   Encounter for care involving renal dialysis
Z51   Encounter for other aftercare

21.2.9.1 Encounter for radiation therapy and chemotherapy
For patients whose encounter is specifically to receive radiation therapy and chemotherapy, codes Z51.0, Encounter for radiotherapy session and Z51.1, Encounter for chemotherapy session for neoplasm, are to be sequenced first, followed by the code for the condition being treated. If a patient receives both radiation and chemotherapy during the same encounter both codes should be used, with either sequenced first.

21.2.10 Donor
Category Z52, Donors of organs and tissues, include the donor codes. They are for use for living individuals who are donating blood or other body tissue. These codes are only for individuals donating for others, not for self donations. They are not for use to identify cadaveric donations.

21.2.11 Counseling
Counseling Z codes are for use when a patient or family member of a patient receives assistance in the aftermath of an illness or injury, or when support is required in coping with family or social problems. These Z codes may be used alone, without a diagnosis code, if the encounter is solely for counseling. They are not necessary for use in conjunction with a diagnosis code when the counseling component of care is integral to standard treatment.

The counseling categories are:

Z69   Encounter for mental health services for victim and perpetrator of abuse
Z70   Counseling related to sexual attitude, behavior and orientation
Z71   Persons encountering health services for other counseling and medical advice, not elsewhere classified

21.2.12 History (of)
There are two types of history (of) codes, personal history and family history. Personal history codes indicate a patient's past medical condition that no longer exists but that has the potential for recurrence, and, therefore, may require continued monitoring.

Family history codes are for use when a patient has a family member(s) who has had a particular disease that causes the patient to be at higher risk of also contracting the disease.

Personal history codes should be used in conjunction with follow-up codes to explain the condition being followed. Family history codes should be used in conjunction with screening codes to explain the need for a test or procedure, if a family history of the condition being screened for is applicable.

Personal history codes are acceptable on any medical record regardless of the reason for the encounter. A personal history or an illness or condition, even if no longer present, is important information that may alter the type of treatment given.

The history (of) categories/codes are:

Z80   Family history of primary malignant neoplasm
Z81   Family history of mental and behavioral disorders
Z82   Family history of certain disabilities and chronic diseases (leading to disablement)
Z83   Family history of other specific disorders
Z84   Family history of other conditions
Z85   Personal history of primary and secondary malignant neoplasm
Z86   Personal history of certain other diseases
Z87   Personal history of other diseases and conditions
Z91.41   Personal history of adult physical and sexual abuse
Z91.49   Other personal history of psychological trauma, not elsewhere classified
Z91.5   Personal history of self-harm
Z92   Personal history of medical treatment

21.2.13 Miscellaneous Z codes

The miscellaneous Z codes capture a number of other health care encounters that do not fall into one of the other general areas. Certain of these codes identify the reason for an encounter that cannot be captured with a diagnosis code, others are for use as additional codes that provide useful information on circumstances that may affect a patient's care and treatment. These codes are generally secondary codes.

The miscellaneous categories/subcategory/codes are:

Z40   Encounter for prophylactic surgery
        A family history code should be used following a code from Z40 to indicate the condition
        for which the patient is seeking prophylactic care.
Z41   Encounters for procedures for purposes other than remedying health state
Z53   Persons encountering health services for specific procedures and treatments, not carried
        out
Z55   Problems related to education and literacy
Z56   Problems related to employment and unemployment
Z57   Occupational exposure to risk-factors
Z58   Problems related to physical environment
Z59   Problems related to housing and economic circumstances
Z60   Problems related to social environment

Z61	Problems related to negative life events in childhood
Z62	Other problems related to upbringing
Z63	Other problems related to primary support group, including family circumstances
Z64	Problems related to certain psychosocial circumstances
Z65	Problems related to other psychosocial circumstances
Z66	Do not resuscitate
Z67	Blood type
Z72	Problems related to lifestyle
Z73	Problems related to life-management difficulty
Z74	Problems related to care-provider dependency
Z75	Problems related to medical facilities and other health care
Z76	Persons encountering health services in other circumstances
Z91.1	Noncompliance with medical treatment and regimen
	Codes from this subcategory are for use when a patient does not take medication or follow therapy as prescribed. It is a distinct concept from poisonings and adverse effects.
Z91.3	Unhealthy sleep-wake schedule
Z91.8	Other specified personal risk-factors, not elsewhere classified

FIRST LISTED

Z codes/categories/that are only acceptable as first listed.

Codes:

Z33.2 Encounter for elective termination of pregnancy

Z51.0 Encounter for radiotherapy session

Z51.1 Encounter for chemotherapy session for neoplasm

   Z51.0 and Z51.1 may be used together on a record, with either one sequenced first, when a patient receives both during the same encounter.

Categories:

Z00 Encounter for general examination without complaint, suspected or reported diagnosis

Z01 Encounter for other special examination without complaint or suspected or reported diagnosis

Z02 Encounter for administrative examination

Z03 Encounter for medical observation for suspected diseases and conditions ruled out

Z04 Encounter for observation for other reasons

Z34 Encounter for supervision of normal pregnancy

Z38 Liveborn infants according to place of birth and type of delivery

Z39 Encounter for maternal postpartum care and examination

Z52 Donors of organs and tissues

FIRST OR ADDITIONAL

Z codes/categories that may be either first listed or additional.

Codes:

Z21 Asymptomatic human immunodeficiency virus [HIV] infection status

Z23 Encounter for immunization

Z51.81 Encounter for therapeutic drug level monitoring

Z51.89 Encounter for other specified aftercare

Categories:

Z08-Z09 Encounters for follow-up examinations

Z11-Z13 Encounters for special screening examinations

Z14 Genetic carrier

Z15 Genetic susceptibility to disease

Z20 Contact with and exposure to communicable diseases

Z22 Carrier of infectious disease

Z23 Encounter for immunization

Z79 Long-term (current) drug therapy

Z85-Z87 Personal history of disease

Z30 Encounter for contraceptive management

Z31   Encounter for procreative management
Z32   Encounter for pregnancy test and instruction
Z36   Encounter for antenatal screening
Z40   Encounter for prophylactic surgery
Z41   Encounter for procedures for purposes other than remedying health state
Z43   Encounter for attention to artificial openings
Z44   Encounter for fitting and adjustment of external prosthetic device
Z45   Encounter for adjustment and management of implanted device
Z46   Encounter for fitting and adjustment of other devices
Z47   Orthopedic aftercare
Z48   Encounter for other surgical aftercare
Z49   Encounter for care involving renal dialysis
Z55-Z65   Persons with potential health hazards related to socioeconomic and psychosocial circumstances
Z69   Encounter for mental health services for victim and perpetrator of abuse
Z70   Counseling related to sexual attitude, behavior and orientation
Z71   Persons encountering health services for other counseling and medical advice, not elsewhere classified
Z72   Problems related to lifestyle
Z73   Problems related to life-management difficulty
Z74   Problems related to care-provider dependency
Z75   Problems related to medical facilities and other health care
Z76   Persons encountering health services in other circumstances
Z89   Acquired absence of limb
Z90   Acquired absence of organs, not elsewhere classified

ADDITIONAL ONLY
    Z codes/subcategories/categories that may be used only as additional codes.

Codes:
Z16   Infection with drug-resistant microorganisms
Z33.1 Pregnant state, incidental
Z51.5 Encounter for palliative care
Z66   Do not resuscitate
Z91.3 Unhealthy sleep-wake schedule
Z91.5 Personal history of self-harm

Subcategories:
Z91.0 Allergy status, other than to drugs and biological substances
Z91.1 Noncompliance with medical treatment and regimen
Z91.4 Personal history of psychological trauma, not elsewhere classified

Categories:

Z28   Immunization not carried out

Z37   Outcome of delivery

Z53   Persons encountering health services for specific procedures and treatment, not carried out

Z67   Blood type

Z80-Z84   Family history of disease

Z86   Allergy status to drugs, medicaments, and biologicals

Z92   Personal history of medical treatment

Z93   Artificial opening status

Z94   Transplanted organ and tissue status

Z95   Presence of cardiac and vascular implants and grafts

Z96   Presence of other functional implants

Z97   Presence of other devices

Z98   Other postsurgical states

Z99   Dependence on enabling machines and devices, not elsewhere classified

Index

Abnormal findings
    on antenatal screening of mother, 128
    on examination of other body fluids, substances, and tissues, 148–49
    fifth characters for presence or absence of, 171
Abortion, elective and spontaneous, 122, 170
Abscess of anal and rectal regions, 98
Accidents
    poisonings, 156, 162
    punctures and lacerations, 72
    transportation, 166
Activity codes, use of for place of injury, 167
Additional codes
    for activity of patient at time of injury, 167
    for alcohol abuse and dependence, 39, 101
    for behavioral disturbance associated with Alzheimer's disease, 58
    for blood alcohol levels, 52
    categories and subcategories used as, 48
    for complications of surgical and medical care, 158–59
    for exposure to environmental tobacco smoke, 39, 94, 95, 101
    for external cause of digestive system disease, 101
    for hepatitis B and C, 39
    for history of tobacco use, 39, 94, 101
    for identifying causation and underlying conditions in diseases of genitourinary system, 119
    for identifying causation in diseases of nervous system, 60
    for identifying injury or poisoning complicating pregnancy, childbirth, or puerperium, 131
    for identifying neoplasm, 131
    for identifying organism in diseases of skin and subcutaneous tissue, 106
    for insulin use, 47
    for manifestations of toxic effects, 156
    for morphology code with behavior code, 39
    for source, place, and intent of burn, 155

    for specifying condition complicating pregnancy, childbirth, or puerperium, 127–28, 129
    for tobacco use and dependence, 39, 94, 101
    for underlying conditions, causative organisms, or neoplasms in musculoskeletal diseases, 113
    for virus in respiratory system diseases, 94
Adnexa, diseases of, 58, 63–65
    additions, deletions, and combinations for, 63–64
    changes in structure for, 65
    changes in terminology for, 64–65
    code ranges and section titles for, 63
    expansions for, 64
    title changes in ICD-10-CM for, 63
Adverse effects, versus poisonings, 155–56
Affective disorders. *See* Mood disorders
Aftercare, encounters for, 172
Alcohol abuse, 52
Allergies, to drugs, medicaments, and biological substances, 175
Alphabetic Index, ICD-10-CM
    abbreviations in, 17–18
    conventions of, 17
    cross-references terms in, 18
    excludes notes in, 14
    includes notes in, 14
    modifiers in, 17
    sections of, 16
    Table of Neoplasms in, 18
Alzheimer's disease, early versus late onset of, 58
Ambulatory care encounters, ICD-10-CM information relevant to, 4
Amebic infections, 29
American Health Information Management Association
    ICD-10-CM viewed as improved code set by, 20
    as one of the Cooperating Parties, 3
    recommendations for code set maintenance of, 20–21

American Hospital Association, as one of the Cooperating Parties, 3
American Public Health Association, 2
Anal fissures and fistula, 98
Angiitis, hypersensitivity, 108
Angina pectoris, 87–88
Antepartum hemorrhage, 130–31
Anxiety disorders, 54–55
Anxiolytic-related disorders, 53
Associated injuries, coding of, 154
Atherosclerosis, 88
Australia, implementation of ICD-10 in, 21, 22

Behavioral and emotional disorders, with onset during childhood and adolescence, 52
Behavioral syndromes, associated with physiological disturbances and physical factors, 55
Behçet's syndrome, 108
Benign mammary dysplasia, 119
Beriberi, 47
Bertillon, Jacques, as author of Bertillon Classification of Causes of Death, 2
Bipolar disease, 53–54
Birth. *See* Childbirth; Delivery
Blood alcohol levels, 6, 52
Blood and blood-forming organs, diseases of, 41–43
    additions, deletions, and combinations for, 41
    code ranges and section titles for, 41
    expansions for, 42–43
    title changes for, 41
Blood pressure, routine encounter for examination of, 171
Bloodtype, 6, 170
Body regions, codes based on, 152
Breast cancer, 39
Bronchitis, acute, 93
Burns and corrosions, 154–55
Bypass graft(s), of transplanted heart, 88

Canada, implementation of ICD-10 in, 22
Cannabis-related disorders, 53
Carcinoma in situ, of breast, 39
Cardiac arrest, physician documentation for, 88
Cardiovascular disease, 87–89
Cataracts, 64–65
Categories, in ICD-10-CM, 6, 8
Centers for Medicare and Medicaid Services, as one of Cooperating Parties, 3
Cerebrovascular disease, late effects of, 73–86
Chagas' disease, 33
Chief financial officer, role of, 25
Childbirth, 121–31
    additions, deletions, and combinations for, 122–24
    code ranges and section titles for, 121

complications of, 127–28
expansions for, 124–31
fourth-character codes for, 125
premature rupture of membranes during, 130
title changes for, 121–22
trauma during, 135, 136
trimester codes for, 6, 121, 123–24, 125–26, 127, 129, 130
Cholelithiasis, 102
Chromosomal abnormalities, 139–43
    additions, deletions, and combinations for, 140
    code ranges and section titles for, 139
    expansions and consolidations for, 140–43
    title changes in ICD-10-CM for, 139
Circulatory system, diseases of, 71–89
    additions, deletions, and combinations for, 71–72
    changes in terminology for, 87–89
    code ranges and section titles for, 71
    expansions for, 72–87
    title changes for, 71
Classification systems, history of, 2–3
Cocaine-related disorders, 53
Code first/use additional code notes, 15
Code sets
    under HIPAA, 19–21
    maintenance of, 20–21
Coded data, uses of, 1–2, 22
Coders. *See* Coding professionals
Codes, grouping of in ICD-10-CM, 5
Codes on Dental Procedures and Nomenclature, Second Edition, 20
Coding Clinic, 3
Coding guidelines, ICD-10-CM, 177
Coding professionals, 3, 25
    shortage of, 23
    training for, 22–23, 25
Coma, Glascow scale for assessing, 149–50
Combination codes, use of in ICD-10-CM, 5, 6
Complications
    of anesthesia, 128–29
    of Crohn's disease, 99
    of diabetes mellitus, 47
    of ectopic and molar pregnancy, 123
    of endocrine procedures, 46
    of malaria, 33
    mechanical, 159–60
    of medical and surgical care, 158–59, 166–67
    of multiple gestation, 129
    of myocardial infarction, 88–89
    of nervous system disorders, 58
    of nonhealing surgical wounds, 152
    postoperative, 5
    of pregnancy, childbirth, or puerperium, 126–27, 127–28, 131
    of procedures, 152
    of procedures on spleen, 43
    related to implants, 159–60
    of respiratory system surgery, 92
    of termination of pregnancy, 122
    of trauma, early, 158

Congenital malformations and deformations, 139–43
    additions, deletions, and combinations for, 140
    code ranges and section titles for, 139
    expansions and consolidations for, 140–43
    title changes in ICD-10-CM for, 139
Connective tissue, diseases of, 98, 107–14
    additions, deletions, and combinations for, 108–9
    code ranges and section titles for, 107
    encounter extensions for, 112–13
    expansions for, 109–14
    title changes for, 107–8
Convalescent care, encounters for, 172
Conventions, in ICD-10-CM, 11–12
Cooperating Parties, 3
Counseling, increased specificity for codes to report, 174–75
Crohn's disease, 99–100
Current Procedural Terminology, Fourth Edition, 20

Decubitus ulcer, 105
Degree of burn, 154
Delivery. *See* Childbirth
Dentofacial anomalies, 98
Dermatitis, 106
Developmental disorders, 52
Diabetes mellitus, 5, 47–48
    complications of, 47
    drug- or chemical-induced, 46
    fourth, fifth, and sixth characters for, 46–48
    manifestations of, 47, 48
    in pregnancy, childbirth, or puerperium, 126
Digestive system, diseases of, 97–102
    additions, deletions, and combinations for, 98
    code ranges and section titles for, 97
    expansions for, 98–102
    title changes in ICD-10-CM for, 97–98
Diverticula of intestine, 102
Documentation assessment, 23
Donation of organ or tissue, Z codes for, 169
Drug- or chemical-induced diabetes mellitus, 46
Drug levels, monitoring of, 175
Drug therapy, long-term, 175
Drugs, poisonings and adverse effects of, 156
Dummy placeholders, 10

E codes, ICD-9-CM
    incorporation of into ICD-10-CM classification, 4
    location of, 162
Ear, diseases of, 58, 67–76
    additions, deletions, and combinations for, 67–69
    code ranges and section titles for, 67
    expansions for, 69–70
    title changes for, 67

Eczema, 106
Encounters, healthcare. *See also* Health services, contact with
    for elective termination of pregnancy, 122, 170
    reasons for, 169–70
    subsequent, 153, 154, 163
Endocrine system, diseases of, 45–49
    additions, deletions, and combinations for, 45–46
    code ranges and section titles for, 45
    expansions for, 47–49
    procedures, complications of, 46
    title changes for, 45
Enteritis, regional, 109
Epilepsy, 60–62
Erythrasma, 104
Etiology of condition, notes for, 15
Eustachian tube disorders, 69
Examinations
    follow-up, 172
    increased specificity for codes related to health, 171–72
    screening, 172
Excludes notes
    for categories and subcategories, 14
    for conditions not otherwise specified, 12
    for drug abuse and drug dependence, 175
    examples of, 14–15
    as expanded in ICD-10-CM, 5
    as ICD-10-CM conventions, 13
    for mental disorders due to known physiological conditions, 56
    modifications in, 11
    for screening examinations, 172
    for symptoms, signs, and abnormal clinical and laboratory findings, 145
    types of, 14
Extensions for categories
    for activity of patient at time of injury, 167
    for fetus having complication code in multiple gestation, 130
    for injuries, poisonings, and other consequences of external causes, 153, 154
    selection of, 10–11
    seventh and final character as, 10, 167
External causes, effects of, 157–58
External causes of morbidity, 161–67
    additions, deletions, and combinations for, 162
    code ranges and section titles for, 161–62
    expansions for, 163–67
    title changes for, 162
Eye, diseases of, 58, 63–65
    additions, deletions, and combinations for, 63–64
    changes in structure for, 65
    changes in terminology for, 64–65
    code ranges and section titles for, 63
    expansions for, 64
    title changes for, 63

Family and personal history, influencing health status, 175
Farr, William, classification of diseases by, 2
Fetal care, 130, 134–35. *See also* Pregnancy
Fields for coding software, expansion to seven alphanumeric characters of, 24
Fifth characters, ICD-9-CM, 5
Foreign bodies, effects of, 154
Forms review, 6
Fractures of bone
    encounter extensions for, 113
    in neoplastic disease, 108
Frostbite, 155

Gangrene, 72, 98–99
Genitourinary system, diseases of, 115–19
    additions, deletions, and combinations for, 116–17
    code ranges and section titles for, 115
    expansions and consolidations for, 117–19
    title changes for, 115
Gestational age, codes based on, 134
Glascow coma scale, 149–50
Gonococcal infection, 28
Goodpasture's syndrome, 108
Gout, 108
Graunt, John, first statistical study of diseases by, 2

Hallucinogen-related disorders, 53
Headache, anesthesia-induced, 129
Health Insurance Portability and Accountability Act, 1, 19–21
Health services, contact for. *See also* Encounters, healthcare
    additions, deletions, and combinations for, 170
    code ranges and section titles for, 169
    expansions for, 170–76
    factors influencing, 169–76
Health status, factors influencing, 169–76
    additions, deletions, and combinations for, 170
    code ranges and section titles for, 169
    expansions for, 170–76
Healthcare Common Procedural Coding System, 20, 24–25
Healthcare encounters. *See* Encounters, healthcare
Healthcare professionals, training in ICD-10-CM for, 23–24
Heart transplants, bypass graft of coronary artery of, 88
Hematoma, 72
Hemorrhage, 72
Hepatitis, 31–32
Hernias, 102
HIV disease, 28
Hodgkin's disease, 39
Human resources personnel, impact of ICD-10-CM on, 25

Hydroxyapatite deposition disease, 108
Hyperemesis gravidarum, 125
Hypertension, 89, 124
Hypnotic-related disorders, 53
Hypoparathyroidism, 47

ICD-9-CM Coordination and Maintenance Committee, role of, 3
ICD-10-AM, 21
ICD-10-CA, 21–22
ICD-9-CM. *See* International Classification of Diseases, Ninth Revision, Clinical Modification
ICD-10-CM. *See* International Classification of Diseases and Related Health Problems, Tenth Revision, Clinical Modification
Immune system, diseases of, 41–43
    additions, deletions, and combinations for, 41
    code ranges and section titles for, 41
    expansions for, 42–43
    title changes for, 41
Impetigo, 105
Implants, complications related to, 159–60
Includes notes
    code modifications in, 11
    for conditions not otherwise specified, 12
    as convention for conditions included in category, 13
    for diseases of digestive system, 101
    for diseases of genitourinary system, 119
    for diseases of musculoskeletal system and connective tissue, 113
    for diseases of nervous system, 60
    for diseases of respiratory system, 94
    for diseases of skin and subcutaneous tissue, 106
    for endocrine, nutritional, and metabolic disorders, 48
    for mental disorders, 56
Infectious diseases, 27–34, 94, 101
Infectious mononucleosis, 32–33
Influenza, with involvement of gastro-intestinal tract, 93
Information systems, impact of ICD-10-CM on, 24–25
Inhalant-related disorders, 53
Initial encounter, extension for, 153, 154, 163
Injuries, 151–60
    additions, deletions, and combinations for, 152
    classification of, 4
    code ranges and section titles for, 151
    expansions for, 153–60
    multiple, 154
    of unspecified body region, 154
International Classification of Causes of Death, 2
International Classification of Diseases, Adapted for Indexing Hospital Records by Diseases and Operations, 2

International Classification of Diseases,
      Adapted for Use in the United States, 2
International Classification of Diseases, Ninth
      Revision, Clinical Modification
   adoption of, 3
   comparison of ICD-10-CM with, 3–6, 136
   HIPAA standards requirements not met by,
      1, 19, 20
   limitations and obsolescence of, 20
   other categories in, 136
   purpose of, 1
International Classification of Diseases and
      Related Health Problems, Tenth
      Revision, Clinical Modification
   Alphabetic Index, 16–18
   benefits of, 4, 20, 24
   code extensions in, 6
   coding guidelines for, 177
   comparison of ICD-9-CM with, 3–6, 136
   data analysts currently using, 24
   decreased specificity in, 170
   development of, 3
   expanded features of, 5
   general structure and characteristics of,
      6–18
   increased specificity of, 20, 23, 42–43, 60,
      69, 73, 138, 147–48, 167, 171–76
   length of compared with ICD-9-CM, 4,
      5–6
   lowercase exes used in, 16
   proposed to meet PPS requirements, 1
   proposed as national code set, 20
   Tabular List, 6–16
   training for, 21–25
   transition to, 24–25
   types of code changes in, 5–6
   vacant categories in, 4
Intestinal infections, 29
Intraoperative and postprocedural complica-
      tions, not elsewhere classified
   and disorders of circulatory system, 72
   and disorders of ear and mastoid process,
      69
   and disorders of genitourinary system, 117
   and disorders of musculoskeletal system,
      109
   and disorders of nervous system, 58
   and disorders of respiratory system, 92
   and disorders of skin and subcutaneous
      tissue, 104
Intubation for anesthesia, during pregnancy,
      129
Irritable bowel syndrome, 100

Jaws, diseases of, 98

Labor. *See* Childbirth
Laboratory findings, abnormal, 145–50
   additions, deletions, and combinations for,
      146–47
   code ranges and section titles for, 145
   expansions for, 147–50
   title changes for, 145–46

Late effects, extension for, 153, 162
Laterality, codes expanded in ICD-10-CM to
      include, 5
   for congenital abnormalities, 142
   for consequences of external causes, 153,
      154
   for diseases of circulatory system, 73
   for diseases of digestive system, 102
   for diseases of ear and mastoid process, 69
   for diseases of eye and adnexa, 64
   for diseases of genitourinary system, 119
   for diseases of musculoskeletal system,
      109, 111–12
   for health services encounters, 172–73
   for injuries and poisonings, 153, 154
Leprosy, 33–34
Lip, diseases of, 101
Lobar pneumonia, 92
Lung abscess, 94

Main terms, in Alphabetic Index, 16
Maintenance of code sets, AHIMA recom-
      mendations for, 20–21
Malaria, 33
Malocclusion, unspecified, 108
Managed care encounters, ICD-10-CM infor-
      mation relevant to, 4
Manifestations
   of acute bronchitis, 93
   of infectious and parasitic diseases, 30–31,
      32
   of diabetes mellitus, 47, 48
   of influenza, 93
   and need for additional code to identify,
      101, 156
   of psoriasis, 106
Mastoid process, diseases of, 58, 67–76
   additions, deletions, and combinations for,
      67–69
   code ranges and section titles for, 67
   expansions for, 69–70
   title changes for, 67
Medicare prospective payment system, 1
Medications, poisonings and adverse effects
      of, 156
Melanoma in situ, 37
Mental and behavioral disorders, 51–56
   additions, deletions, and combinations for,
      52
   changes in directions for, 55–56
   changes in terminology for, 55
   code ranges and section titles for, 51
   expansions and consolidations for, 52–55
   due to known physiological conditions, 56
   due to psychoactive substance use, 52–53
   nonpsychotic, 54–55
   title changes for, 51–52
Mental retardation, 55–56
Metabolic disorders, 45–49
   additions, deletions, and combinations for,
      45–46
   code ranges and section titles for, 45
   expansions for, 47–49
   title changes for, 45

Migraine, 59
Mineral deficiency, 48
Modifiers, use of in Alphabetic Index, 17
Mononeuropathies, 62
Mood disorders, 53
Morbidity. *See* External causes of morbidity
Multiple gestations, 129–30
Musculoskeletal system, diseases of, 98,
   107–14
   additions, deletions, and combinations for,
      108–9
   code ranges and section titles for, 107
   encounter extensions for, 112–13
   expansions for, 109–14
   title changes for, 107–8
Myocardial infarction, 88–89

National Center for Classification in Health
   (Australia), 21
National Center for Health Statistics, 3
National code set, ICD-10-CM proposed as,
   20
National Drug Codes, 20
NEC, abbreviation used in Alphabetic Index,
   17–18
Neoplasm, malignant
   of esophagus, 36
   follow-up examinations for, 172
   of kidney and other and unspecified
      organs, 38
   personal history of, 175
   of pleura, 36–37
   during pregnancy, 131
   of retroperitoneum and peritoneum, 36
Neoplasms, 35–39
   additions, deletions, and combinations for,
      36–37
   code ranges and section titles for, 35
   expansions and consolidations for, 37–39
   table for, 18
   title changes for, 35–36
   of uncertain behavior, 39
Nervous system, diseases of, 57–62
   additions, deletions, and combinations for,
      57–58
   changes in terminology for, 60–62
   code ranges and section titles for, 57
   expansions for, 58–60
   title changes for, 57
Neuropathy
   hereditary, 116
   inflammatory and toxic, 59
Newborns
   affected by noxious influences, 134
   low-birth-weight, 135
   preterm, 135
Nicotine dependence, 53
Nodular prostate, 117
Nonmedicinal substances, toxic effects of,
   156
Not elsewhere classified, use of in category or
   code title, 12, 17–18

Not otherwise specified, 12
Notes, use of in ICD-10-CM, 13–15
   Includes notes, 13–15
   Excludes notes, 13–15
Nutritional disorders, 45–49
   additions, deletions, and combinations for,
      45–46
   code ranges and section titles for, 45
   expansions for, 47–49
   title changes for, 45

Obstetrics, need for indication of patient's
   trimester for, 5. *See also* Childbirth;
   Pregnancy; Puerperium
Obstructed labor, 131
Official Coding Guidelines, 3
Opioid-related disorders, 53
Oral mucosa, diseases of, 101
Osteoarthritis, 114
Osteomalacia, adult, 108
Osteomyelitis, subacute, 109
Osteoporosis, with current pathological frac-
   ture, 112, 113
Otitis media, 69
Outcome of delivery code, 131
Ovaries, hyperstimulation of, 116
Other categories, use of in ICD-9-CM, 136

Parasitic diseases, 27–34
Parentheses, use of in ICD-10-CM, 11–12
Patella, dislocation of, 108
Patient care, importance of physician docu-
   mentation for, 23
Perinatal period, conditions originating in,
   133–38
Peripheral arteriovenous aneurysms, 140
Personality and behavior, adult disorders of,
   52
Pharyngitis, acute, 94
Physicians
   documentation by, 23, 88, 124, 138, 149
   training in ICD-10-CM for, 23
Place of occurrence, of injuries, 167
Pneumonia, 92
Poisonings, 151–60
   accidental or unintentional, 162
   additions, deletions, and combinations for,
      152
   adverse effects versus, 155–56
   code ranges and section titles for, 151
   expansions for, 153–60
   intent of, 157
Poliomyelitis, 34
Polyarteritis nodosa, 108
Postcardiotomy syndrome, 72
Postmastectomy lymphedema syndrome, 72
Postoperative hypertension, 72
Postprocedural conditions, ICD-10-CM codes
   for, 6
Pregnancy, 121–31
   additions, deletions, and combinations for,
      122–24

code ranges and section titles for, 121
complications of, 126–28
expansions for, 124–31
fourth-character codes for, 125
high-risk, supervision of, 123–24
title changes for, 121–22
trimester codes for, 6, 121, 123–24, 125–26, 127, 129, 130
Prospective payment systems, ICD-10-CM proposed for use with, 1
Prostheses, complications and reactions to, 159–60
Proteinuria, 124
Psoriasis, manifestations of, 106
Psychotic disorders, nonmood, 55. *See also* Behavioral and mental disorders
Puerperium
    additions, deletions, and combinations for, 122–24
    code ranges and section titles for, 121
    complications of, 127–28
    conditions arising during, 121–31
    expansions for, 124–31
    fourth-character codes for, 125
    title changes for, 121–22
Pulmonary embolism, 88

Radon, exposure to, 162
Reason for encounter, Z codes for, 169
Reduction defects, of upper and lower limbs, 142–43
Reimbursement systems, 1, 25
Renal failure, chronic, 118
Reproduction, healthcare encounters related to, 170
Respiratory system, diseases of, 91–95
    additions, deletions, and combinations for, 92
    changes in terminology for, 95
    code ranges and section titles for, 91
    expansions for, 93–95
    title changes for, 91
Rheumatoid arthritis, juvenile, 109
Rubrics. *See* ICD-10-CM, categories in

Salivary glands, diseases of, 101
Schizophrenia, 55
Screening examinations, 172
Sedative-related disorders, 53
Sepsis, 31
Septisemia. *See* Sepsis
Sequela, use of extensions for
    for external causes of morbidity, 163
    of injuries and poisonings, 153, 154
    of other consequences of external causes, 153, 154
    and late effects, 162
Signs and symptoms, 145
Sinusitis, acute, 92
Skeletal fluorosis, 108
Skin, diseases of, 103–6
    additions, deletions, and combinations for, 104

code ranges and section titles for, 103
    expansions for, 104–6
    title changes for, 103–4
Sleep disorders, 55
Smallpox, 34
Socioeconomic and psychosocial circumstances, influencing health status, 173–74
Software vendors, 23, 24
Somatoform disorders, 54–55
Spleen, intraoperative and postprocedural complications of, 43
Square brackets, use of in ICD-10-CM, 11
Stimulant-related disorders, 53
Stomatitis, 101
Stress fracture, encounters for, 113
Stress incontinence, 116
Stress-related mental disorders, 54–55
Subarachnoid hemorrhage, nontraumatic, 72–73, 88
Subcategories
    as divisions of categories in ICD-9-CM, 8–10
    expanded to fifth and sixth characters, 49
    titles of, 5
Subcutaneous tissue, diseases of, 103–6
    additions, deletions, and combinations for, 104
    code ranges and section titles for, 103
    expansions for, 104–6
    title changes in ICD-10-CM for, 103–4
Substance-related disorders, 53, 175
Symptoms and signs, 145–50
    additions, deletions, and combinations for, 146–47
    code ranges and section titles for, 145
    expansions for, 147–50
    title changes for, 145–46
Syphilis, 28
Systemic antibiotics, poisonings and adverse effects of, 156

Table of Neoplasms, 18
Tabular List, 6–16
    conventions followed in, 11–16
    structure of chapters in, 7–11
Tobacco use and dependence, 53
Tongue, diseases of, 101
Tonsillitis, acute, 93
Transportation accidents, 166
Trauma, early complications of, 158
Tuberculosis, 29–30
Tympanic membrane, perforation of, 69
Tympanosclerosis, 70
Typhoid fever, 29

Ulcerative colitis, 109
Ulcers, 101, 105
Umbilical hernia, 98–99

Underlying disease, coding of, 60, 69, 94, 106
Underlying neoplasm, coding of, 60
United States Public Health Service, 2
Urethritis, nonspecific, 116
Use additional code notes, 15

V codes, ICD-9-CM
    incorporation into main ICD-10-CM classification of, 4
    Z codes compared with, 170
Vaccinations, prophylactic, 169, 172

Vagina, noninflammatory disorders of, 119
Vesicoureteral-reflux, with and without hydroureter, 116
Virus, identification for respiratory system diseases of, 94
Volume depletion, 46
Vomiting, in pregnancy, 125

World Health Organization, 2, 3–4

X-ray reports, 151

AHIMA Certification:
Your Valuable Career Asset

AHIMA offers a variety of credentials whether you're just starting out in the health information management (HIM) field, are an advanced coding professional, or play an important privacy or security role at your facility. Employers are looking for your commitment to the field and a certain competency level. AHIMA credentials help you stand out from the crowd of resumes.

- ✔ Registered Health Information Administrator (RHIA)/Registered Health Information Technician (RHIT)
- ✔ Certified Coding Associate (CCA), entry-level
- ✔ Certified Coding Specialist (CCS), advanced
- ✔ Certified Coding Specialist—Physician-based (CCS-P), advanced
- ✔ Certified in Healthcare Privacy (CHP)
- ✔ Certified in Healthcare Security (CHS), Offered by HIMSS through AHIMA
- ✔ Certified in Healthcare Privacy and Security (CHPS)–AHIMA in conjunction with HIMSS

In recent AHIMA-sponsored research groups, healthcare executives and recruiters cited three reasons for preferring credentialed personnel:

1. Assurance of current knowledge through continued education
2. Possession of field-tested experience
3. Verification of base level competency

AHIMA is a premier organization for HIM professionals, with more than 45,000 members nationwide. AHIMA certification carries a strong reputation for quality—the requirements for our certification are rigorous.

AHIMA exams are computer-based and available throughout the year.

Make the right move...pair your degree and experience with AHIMA certification to maximize your career possibilities.

For more information on AHIMA credentials and how to sit for the exams, you can either visit our Web site at www.ahima.org/certification, send an e-mail to **certdept@ahima.org**, or call **(800) 335-5535**.

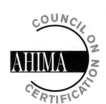

Join AHIMA and Gain "Insider Knowledge"

The Exclusive Province of AHIMA Members!

Nowhere else will you find the kind of "Insider Knowledge" you can acquire from our highly active membership of more than 45,000 health information management (HIM) professionals! Combine this depth of exclusive knowledge with your fresh ideas and new perspectives and you've come up with a winning combination, one that will lead you in new directions in professionalism and career growth.

When you join AHIMA, your most prominent benefit is "Insider Knowledge." All other benefits relate back to the knowledge you gain. Here are just a few areas where "Insider Knowledge" helps you thrive:

Workplace solutions: From columns on HIPAA, coding, and best practices in the award-winning *Journal of AHIMA*, to *Advantage* e-alerts on industry news, to the *Advantage* newsletter, and more, you get the kind of insider knowledge you won't find elsewhere… the kind of knowledge that puts you ahead of the competition.

Career growth: From certification to education, AHIMA membership offers you exclusive benefits for making the most of your career by helping you gain the knowledge to excel and lead.

Networking: Where else can you get access to more than 45,000 of your professional peers? Our unique virtual network, Communities of Practice, gives you the ability to search for and join forces with like-minded professionals to solve problems and strategize to make the most of your career!

Membership in AHIMA is a bargain. Active or associate membership is only $135 per year, and student membership is just $20 per year.

Need more reasons to join? Go to www.ahima.org/membership to see how joining America's premier HIM Association benefits you.

Insider Knowledge… Join Today and Gain Instant Access!

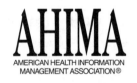

AMERICAN HEALTH INFORMATION
MANAGEMENT ASSOCIATION®

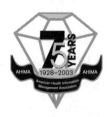

Look for These Quality AHIMA Publications at Bookstores, Libraries, and Online

Clinical Coding Workout: Practice Exercises for Skill Development
AHIMA Coding Products and Services Team

Applying Inpatient Coding Skills under Prospective Payment
Vickie L. Rogers, MS, RHIA

Basic CPT/HCPCS Coding
Gail I. Smith, MA, RHIA, CCS-P

Basic Healthcare Statistics for Health Information Management Professionals
Karen G. Youmans, MPA, RHIA, CCS

Basic ICD-9-CM Coding
Lou Ann Schraffenberger, MBA, RHIA, CCS, CCS-P

CPT/HCPCS Coding and Reimbursement for Physician Services
Lynne Kuehn, RHIA, CCS-P, FAHIMA, and LaVonne Wieland, RHIT

Documentation and Reimbursement for Home Care and Hospice Programs
Prinny Rose Abraham, RHIT, CPHQ

Documentation for Ambulatory Care
AHIMA Ambulatory Care Section

Documentation Requirements for the Acute Care Patient Record
Barbara A. Glondys, RHIA

Quality and Performance Improvement in Healthcare: A Tool for Programmed Learning
Patricia Shaw, MEd, RHIA;
Chris Elliot, MS, RHIA;
Polly Isaacson, RHIA, CPHQ;
and Elizabeth Murphy, MEd, RN

Effective Management of Coding Services
Edited by Lou Ann Schraffenberger, MBA, RHIA, CCS, CCS-P

Finance Principles for the Health Information Manager
Rose T. Dunn, RHIA, CPA, FHFMA

Health Information Management Compliance: A Model Program for Healthcare Organizations
Sue Prophet, RHIA, CCS

Health Information Management Technology: An Applied Approach
Edited by Merida L. Johns, PhD, RHIA

ICD-9-CM Coding for Long-Term Care
Edited by Reesa Gottschalk, RHIA

ICD-9-CM Diagnostic Coding and Reimbursement for Physician Services
Anita C. Hazelwood, MLS, RHIA, FAHIMA
and Carol A. Venable, MPH, RHIA

Reimbursement Methodologies for Healthcare Services
Edited by Lolita M. Jones, RHIA, CCS

Health Information Management: Concepts, Principles, and Practice
Kathleen M. LaTour, MA, RHIA,
and Shirley Eichenwald, MBA, RHIA, CPHIMS

Need to Know More?

Textbook details and easy ordering are available online on the AHIMA Web site at **www.ahima.org.** Click on "Professional Development." In addition to textbooks, AHIMA offers other educational products such as online training programs and audio seminars. For textbook content questions contact **publications@ahima.org,** and for sales information contact **resources@ahima.org.**

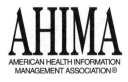
AMERICAN HEALTH INFORMATION MANAGEMENT ASSOCIATION®

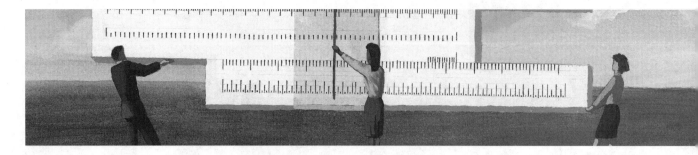

Medical Coding Accuracy: The Key to Profitable Healthcare Provider Operation

AHIMA's Web-based *Coding Assessment and Training Solutions* Maintains and Increases the Proficiency of Coding Staff

The American Health Information Management Association's (AHIMA's) *Coding Assessment and Training Solutions* is a uniquely customizable training remedy.

Use this program to target and train in areas specific to your area of need. We have modules covering specialties from pregnancy and childbirth to digestive disease and services.

Coding Assessment and Training Solutions propels coding professionals toward greater standards of achievement. Through the use of this program, medical coders will:

- Increase the accuracy of clinical coding that affects reimbursement

- Reduce the occurrence of bounceback claims due to coding errors

- Increase reliability of data elements used for disease management and decision support

- Increase the competency level of both new and experienced coders

For more information, visit our Web site at http://campus.ahima.org, and click on "Catalog".

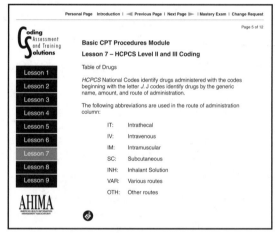

Clear and concise course content is delivered in an intuitive format to facilitate straightforward lesson progression.

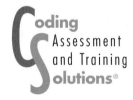

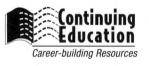

Visit our online campus to learn more about our other e-learning products.

http://campus.ahima.org

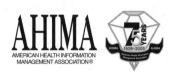